· ·

Making the Connection Between Brain and Behavior

Making the Connection Between Brain and Behavior

COPING WITH

Parkinson's Disease

Second Edition

Joseph H. Friedman, MD

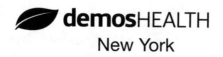

demosHEALTH

New York

Visit our website at www.demoshealth.com

ISBN: 978-1-936303-53-3
e-book ISBN: 978-1-61705-175-3

Acquisitions Editor: Julia Pastore
Compositor: diacriTech

Medical information provided by Demos Health, in the absence of a visit with a health care professional, must be considered as an educational service only. This book is not designed to replace a physician's independent judgment about the appropriateness or risks of a procedure or therapy for a given patient. Our purpose is to provide you with information that will help you make your own health care decisions.

The information and opinions provided here are believed to be accurate and sound, based on the best judgment available to the authors, editors, and publisher, but readers who fail to consult appropriate health authorities assume the risk of injuries. The publisher is not responsible for errors or omissions. The editors and publisher welcome any reader to report to the publisher any discrepancies or inaccuracies noticed.

Library of Congress Cataloging-in-Publication Data
Friedman, Joseph H.
  Making the connection between brain and behavior : coping with Parkinson's disease / Joseph H. Friedman.—2nd ed.
    p. ; cm.
  Includes index.
  ISBN 978-1-936303-53-3—ISBN 978-1-61705-175-3 (e-book)
  I. Title.
  [DNLM: 1. Parkinson Disease—complications.   2. Parkinson Disease—physiopathology.   3. Caregivers—psychology.   4. Parkinson Disease—therapy.   WL 359]
  RC382
  616.8'33—dc23
                          2013010001

Special discounts on bulk quantities of Demos Health books are available to corporations, professional associations, pharmaceutical companies, health care organizations, and other qualifying groups. For details, please contact:

Special Sales Department
Demos Medical Publishing, LLC
11 West 42nd Street, 15th Floor
New York, NY 10036
Phone: 800-532-8663 or 212-683-0072
Fax: 212-941-7842
E-mail: specialsales@demosmedpub.com

Printed in the United States of America by McNaughton & Gunn Inc.
15 16 17 / 5 4 3 2 1

*My patients, whose courage, resilience, and fortitude
are a never-ending source of inspiration*

and to:

*Meg, whose loyalty, sensitivity, capability, intelligence, work
ethic, and devotion has been the foundation of our efforts to
improve the treatment of Parkinson's disease.*

*"How do you know it's a hallucination,
if you see them outside your house?"*

*"Well, every morning I see a group of nuns,
wearing habits, building me a deck."*

Contents

Foreword

A s a neurologist, I was trained to think of Parkinson's disease as the prototypical movement disorder. As a patient, I learned it was much more. It is an often debilitating cognitive behavioral disorder which also has sensory and physical manifestations.

Quality of life for people living with Parkinson's disease depends largely on better management of these behavioral issues. In *Making the Connection Between Brain and Behavior: Coping with Parkinson's Disease*, Dr. Friedman focuses on these aspects in great detail. He also focuses on the interactions between the person living with Parkinson's, his or her social environment, and the consequences to the family unit.

This book is not only for Parkinson's patients and their caregivers, but also for their physicians. The good physicians will strive to master the slowness, the rigidity, the tremor, and the postural imbalance. The excellent physicians, like Dr. Joseph Friedman, will focus on the whole patient—including the psyche—the depression, the delusional thinking, the dementia, and the common demoralization. These can dishearten and undermine even the strongest among us. But there is hope to be found in this book.

The publication of *Making the Connection Between Brain and Behavior: Coping with Parkinson's Disease* is a source of great hope to all who battle the "shaking palsy" every day of their lives.

Lee Coleman Krapin, MD
Attending Physician and Neurology Consultant,
Albany County Nursing Home and
Ann Lee Home, Albany, NY.
Commander, Medical Corps, U.S. Navy (Retired)

Preface

This book is intended for lay people with Parkinson's disease (PD) as well as those who care about someone with PD. It is written at a level for people who have little or no scientific or medical knowledge.

I have tried not to water down the material. I hope that it is not too simple for sophisticated nonphysicians in medical fields, or too technical for others in nonmedical fields. Technical terms are used but are explained. There is a glossary. Vignettes will be used to illustrate common problems. There are only general discussions of treatment approaches because these vary so much from individual to individual. Practical advice and common sense are my guiding principles. I hope to address all the common behavioral problems that PD patients and their families encounter.

This book is intended to be a source of practical information. It will hopefully not contain inflammatory advice. All opinions of the author will be clearly stated as such, to avoid conflating my own ideas with those of the general PD community. If there are opposing opinions, I will mention them.

· ·

Introduction to the First Edition

All serious diseases affect families and a network of individuals. It is much like the hub of a wheel. Cancer, heart disease, ulcerative colitis, emphysema, psychiatric disorders, and an untold number of other conditions alter interpersonal dynamics in a large number of ways. The person's independence may be affected. One day the family head, the main bread winner, may suddenly find him- or herself to be in need of assistance instead of the other way around. The person everyone counted on suddenly needs help.

When the tables turn the stresses can be enormous. And while many of these stresses may be obvious, such as for a single parent who supports three children and develops PD, just as the oldest is getting ready to apply to college, some can be subtle or downright surprising. Some of the PD patients who had deep brain stimulation became so much better after their surgeries that they went from being almost completely dependent on their spouse, to being completely independent and sometimes well enough to return to work. And while that is obviously a wonderful miracle, some families actually fell apart as a result.

The caregiver whose main role in life was defined by the ill PD patient suddenly has nothing to do, no role in the family, no one to supervise. All of a sudden, he or she is an "empty nester." While such problems are uncommon, I mention this to show that people's responses to changes may not be predictable. Behavior is a complex thing, and we all need humility in attempting to deal with it. Nevertheless, there is a lot we do know about behavioral changes in PD, although there is even more to learn.

This book represents a distillation of more than three decades of experience with PD patients and their families. I wrote this out of a sense of obligation, partly from my love and respect for my patients and their supporters, partly because I love my work, and partly because I think that my own personal intellectual journey depicts a tale that is educational for patients as well as for doctors.

As I tell my patients: When you get older you don't get any smarter, but if you're lucky and you work hard, you may get wiser. I began my PD career as a strong believer that PD was a disease of the motor system and everything else was of secondary importance. James Parkinson himself noted that "the senses and intellect" were untouched. That turned out to be wrong. Behavioral issues are as much a part of the disease as tremor. But, more importantly, I've come to recognize the role I play in my patients' lives. From the occasional letter of thanks that I've received from family members after a patient died, I learned that simply being there was my central function.

I was the doctor who received the call about some new ailment. Was it due to PD or was it due to something else? I was the one who reassured patients that they weren't "crazy" because they were seeing children in the backyard who weren't there. I was the one who told them that the aching discomfort in the shoulder or the back was due to PD or that the stabbing pain in the abdomen was not due to the PD. I could reassure them that they were doing well and that we would work together.

The fact that I was part of the "team," that I was "on their side," that I could put their personal journeys into a general context was of the greatest importance. In their worlds, they were unique. When patients touched base with me they renewed acquaintanceship with the wider world of PD. Their symptoms were validated. "Oh, so other PD patients have that problem too." And I learned that my knowledge about drugs and how to manage the various clinical motor problems was actually less important than simply being an anchor in a stormy sea. I learned that emotional problems were as "real" as shuffling and falling. I learned that too many of my colleagues spent their time on the motor aspects of PD, that is, the movement and balance problems, and not enough on the behavior issues, which were often even more troubling.

When we think of a "disease" we usually think we know what we're talking about, but when we look at people with PD we see a rather wide spectrum of problems. Some people have tremor while some don't. Some are stooped, some freeze, some can't talk, and so on. James Parkinson is justifiably famous because he saw the threads that connected all of these disorders and thought they were different manifestations of the same underlying condition.

What most doctors, even neurologists, don't realize is that while we use motor dysfunction to diagnose PD, it is actually the behavioral problems that cause the most devastating consequences of this illness. It took me many years to recognize this, and when patients and families face these behavioral problems they feel surprised and alone because they always thought that PD caused tremors, and not much else.

Published studies have clearly shown that the most important problems causing nursing home placement of the PD patient is not slowness or the inability to walk. They are psychiatric. Similarly, the most stressful problems for caretakers are behavioral, not motor. It is more stressful to care for a PD patient who can walk independently but has behavioral problems than a PD patient who is wheelchair bound but without behavior problems.

The reader must keep in mind that all people have unique behaviors and that not everything that "goes wrong" or changes is due to the Parkinson's disease. The reader must also be aware that our understanding is in flux. It took 20 years before anyone made a connection between gambling and dopamine agonists. It took over 150 years before REM sleep disorder was recognized in PD. What are we missing today?

Twenty years ago there was very little written about the behavioral aspects of PD. Some authorities wrote about depression, but whole problem areas were virtually terra incognita. Twenty years ago the first papers on treating psychosis appeared. Fifteen years ago the sleep problems of PD were first explored. Dementia, the most difficult and devastating of all the problems, has only been a significant research target for the past decade. Naming and identifying a problem makes it easier to discuss. Confirming that behavioral changes are part of the disease process make it more likely that patients and families will reveal these changes to their doctors, just as they ask about their various aches and pains and changes in bowel and bladder and the various other bodily functions.

There is no reason to read this book in the order presented. Most people with PD will find that only some of the chapters apply to them. Few will find that all of the chapters apply.

I will be happy to hear from readers with their suggestions for modifying future editions, should there be a strong enough interest to justify writing one. I am confident that much of what I write will become dated in a few years, but since much of this book reflects common sense, that part will not go out of date.

· ·

Introduction to the Second Edition

Since the first edition of *Making the Connection Between Brain and Behavior* was published in 2008, I have received a lot of positive feedback. And, thankfully, there has been no negative feedback. This book has helped many people and by updating and expanding it for the second edition, I hope to help many more.

Each chapter has been revised. In some cases the changes were minute; in others they were extensive. I've also added three chapters (16–18) and two appendices (C, D). The new chapters address three of the most common issues I am currently asked about now. The appendices do not address the behavioral aspects of PD, but I wrote them in the belief that they would be helpful to people struggling with the difficulties of PD, and they were widely distributed in the PD community in the United States. The chapters that were updated, unfortunately, did not require as much revision as I would have wished. I regret to tell you that advances in treatment have been modest since the first edition. On the other hand there has been a dramatic increase in the appreciation that neurologists now have for the behavioral aspects of PD, and all knowledgeable neurologists are aware that behavior changes are as much a part of PD as the changes in movement. This is due to the increasing numbers of scientific papers addressing the behavioral problems of PD, underscoring their importance, and the greater attention these areas have been getting in the medical community.

Advances in clinical medicine require interest, intelligence, and resources. Creativity is helpful, but not necessarily required. There are many talented, interested, and intelligent doctors keen on improving the treatment of PD. Unfortunately, resources are limited. There are few funds available to subsidize the very expensive clinical trials required for testing new treatments, and, you may be amazed to read this, but we often have trouble finding PD patients willing to participate in research studies. In a study of antidepressants in PD that ended earlier this year, major academic centers had difficulty recruiting even two subjects per year. The study was successful, but had to stop only halfway through due to the problem of getting PD patients to volunteer. This is not a unique situation.

So, there have been no "breakthroughs" since the first edition yet progress has been made. We have a much better grasp on the impulse control disorders associated with dopamine agonists. The neurological community has a much greater understanding of the importance of behavioral aspects of PD, both in terms of their frequency and in terms of their importance in quality of life. Patients and their families are better informed and demand better care. We finally have data demonstrating that depression can be treated successfully in PD.

But many things are still left to do. The battle goes on. For those who live the battle every day, it is hoped that this small contribution will at least lighten the load a little.

. . . .

Making the Connection
Between
Brain and Behavior

Overview

Behaviors in people develop in complex, poorly understood ways. From studies of patients with Parkinson's disease (PD), we know that certain types of behaviors are considerably more common in PD patients than in the general population, forcing us to conclude that these behaviors are related to the disease. In some cases the problem is part of the disease, due directly to the involvement of certain brain cells. In other cases the problem may be due to the physical disability and represents a "reactive" process, that is, the mind's reaction to having the disease in the first place. An overview is provided of some of the major topics concerning behaviors in persons with PD.

We all see the world differently. Our experiences are unique and ever-changing so that our behavior changes as we mature. Some individuals seem to change less than others, which is usually perceived as a negative thing, a sign of inflexibility, as if the person has failed to adapt to changes in the environment. We like to think that age produces wisdom, as experience increasingly alters our perceptions of the world.

Sometimes there is little adaptation. We see older people developing relatively fixed behaviors that don't change from year to year. Their schedule becomes their religion. But behavior is always in some degree of flux, if for no other reason than the environment is always changing.

PD is a defining trait. Most people do not have it, so that having it puts one in a minority and thus singles one out as being different from one's peers, friends, and relatives. It colors the lives of both the patients and their families. One cannot choose to *not* change. Some changes that occur may be nonspecific, or even just appear with normal aging, but some changes occur so frequently that doctors who specialize in PD think there is probably a connection either with PD itself, the medications used to treat PD, or possibly just the uncertainty of the future due to the vagaries of how PD progresses.

Most PD experts would say that behavioral changes that occur during this disease are due to both primary brain changes and the patient's reaction to having the disease. The basic personality of the patient determines how the various disabilities of PD, the sudden change in one's future plans, and the insecurity of the future affect the person's psyche. For example, will the person, faced with a disability or an attention-grabbing tremor, "give in" by withdrawing from the world, or "fight back" by refusing to compromise his or her lifestyle? Will someone work as long as possible, or get disability as soon as possible? Will the onset of PD trigger a rush to do all the things planned for retirement for fear of not being able to do them when the planned time arrives, or will it trigger the opposite, the giving up of all plans and various vacations or adventures? Optimists behave in one way, pessimists in another. "Realists" react in one way, and "deniers" bury their heads and act as if there is nothing wrong.

There are a number of behavioral issues that occur in PD, some of which are unique to PD, or almost so, while others may be fairly generic across the range of neurological or even just progressive, incurable, potentially disabling medical disorders. To make a point and be very specific, let me briefly introduce two fascinating behavioral issues in PD, one of which is relatively specific to PD, and the other of which is seen in virtually all medical disorders.

Rapid eye movement (REM) sleep behavior disorder (RBD) (see Chapter 12) is seen almost only in PD or dementia with Lewy bodies (see Chapter 7), or in multisystem atrophy, which are all closely related disorders. In RBD, patients, typically male, act out their dreams by punching or choking their bed partners. This is due to PD and is not a drug-related behavior. It is due to specific pathological changes in the brain. It is specific to only a small number of diseases.

Fatigue is very common in PD, causing more disability than most other common symptoms. Yet fatigue also affects almost all patients with significant anemia, congestive heart failure, cancers of all types, hypothyroid disease, sleep disorders, lupus erythematosis, multiple sclerosis, and a multitude of other disorders. Fatigue often occurs, for no understandable reason, in otherwise healthy people, but is much more common and often more severe in almost every medical, neurological, and psychiatric disorder, with the lone exception of mania. Still, fatigue is an integral part of the PD syndrome. Patients usually did not have it before they developed PD, and in some cases fatigue developed long before patients realized there was anything else wrong with them other than a lack of energy.

So, PD patients may have very unusual and specific problems, such as RBD, or commonplace problems that many other people also have. Just because fatigue is common to many disorders does not mean that it is not also "specific" to PD, by which I mean that it is associated with a variety of other symptoms, may have a different cause, and may respond to different forms of treatment than fatigue in other disorders.

Some of the behavioral changes in PD are due to medications, but most are not.

The two most troublesome complications of PD are dementia and psychosis. Dementia is not caused by the drugs used, although they certainly may contribute. By dementia, we mean an irreversible process that results in impaired memory and thinking. About 30% of

PD patients have impaired memory and thought processing, which we believe is part of the disease process and is not due to medications. With time, the chance of this developing increases. While these changes are different from those seen in Alzheimer's disease, there are some similarities. Psychosis is the term given to a major change in thinking, in which hallucinations and delusions are common, often causing impaired reality testing. This problem is generally caused by the anti-PD medications, but dementia may bring with it some of these problems as well, causing an increased difficulty in the treatment, as you will see in Chapter 7.

Sleepiness and sleep disorders are probably as common as constipation in PD. Excessive daytime sleepiness may arise from untreated PD or as a complication of some of the PD medications, particularly the dopamine agonists, pramipexole (Mirapex), ropinerole (Requip), and rotigotine (Neupro).

Depression, anxiety, apathy, and fatigue are probably the most common of all behavioral aspects of PD, yet little is known about any of them. Depression, anxiety, and fatigue are common in the general population and even more so in any population of sick people. But these are serious problems to the PD patient because they have such a deleterious effect on quality of life. Depression is usually treatable, but there are virtually no data to guide the treatment of anxiety, fatigue, or apathy.

There has been much discussion, but very little research, about the so-called parkinsonian personality, by which is meant a relatively rigid, obsessive, and humorless person who does little for fun and lives out the "Protestant ethic" of a life filled with hard work. Despite more than 60 years of hypothesizing, we still do not know how much of these beliefs are myths and how much may be true.

A 65-year-old woman moved to a new house to better accommodate her disability. She developed problems sleeping through the night, depression, and severe kyphoscoliosis (a spine condition). Treatment with one selective serotonin reuptake inhibitor (SSRI) antidepressant was not very helpful, and something was prescribed to help her sleep. She started seeing a psychologist who provided "talk therapy" and also suggested a change from one SSRI to another. Her PD medications were not changed. As she began to sleep through the night, her depression and anxiety improved and her posture became almost erect. She got her energy back, stopped having backaches, and felt like a new person. Even though her medications often wore off, she did not develop a terribly stooped posture anymore. Her PD support group friends continually asked her, "What did your doctor put you on to help your posture so much?"

This is a wonderful and true example of how the behavioral and motor aspects of PD intermingle. Very often if one aspect of the person's situation improves, other aspects do as well. In this case it was unclear to the patient and her doctors whether the improved sleep helped the depression and anxiety, whether the improved depression helped the sleep and anxiety, or whether the improved anxiety helped the sleep and depression—but the one thing that all agreed on was that whatever improved her sleep, depression, and anxiety helped her posture since there was no change in her anti-PD medications.

A 68-year-old man with a 10-year history of PD suffered from uncontrollable clinical fluctuations, with uncomfortable or disabling dyskinesias during about 25% of the day, and severe "off" periods for another 25% of the day. He refused to consider deep brain stimulation. A variety of medication adjustments were not helpful. On one office visit, he reported that he had been on vacation for two weeks and during that time he had virtually no off periods and the dyskinesias were not troubling. In fact, he was able to use a ladder to climb on and off a boat and go sailing without any problem, something he had been unable to do for the previous two years. When he returned home to Rhode Island, however, he

was as bad as he had ever been, although he had made no change
in his medication regimen.

The influence of psychological effects is profound in PD. Tremors resolve with relaxation and worsen with stress. People freeze if they think others are looking at them. People who freeze may unfreeze if they step over lines on the ground. One of my teachers used to say that the first person out of a chair in an emergency is the patient with PD who can't get out of the chair if you ask him to.

A recently recognized set of problems arising from the treatment of PD includes compulsive activities, particularly gambling, but also shopping, hypersexual activity, eating, and many other things as well (see Chapter 11).

The final point to make in this overview is that the more we study PD the more we learn, much of which is so obvious in retrospect that we often wonder how we were *not* able to see it for so long. Now that PD is increasingly recognized as a neurobehavioral disorder, and not just a movement disorder, we see these behavioral aspects receive increased attention and better treatment.

If you have a behavioral problem that you have not yet discussed with your doctor, you should do so. You will not know if it is part of PD until you ask. You may be the one to get your doctor to recognize that this problem is, in fact, a common problem in PD that has simply gone unrecognized. Helping your doctor to recognize the problem in you may alert him or her to the same problem in other PD patients.

2

. . . .

Personality

We all know what is meant when we talk about someone's personality, but it is not so easy to define. Many doctors have thought that there is a "Parkinson's personality"—that PD patients tend to be similar to one another in a particular way, and that this is either part of the disease or a reaction to it. Generally, PD patients have been described as serious, unwilling to take risks, somewhat inflexible, hard working, obsessive, and introspective. All of the studies on the topic of personality have reported conflicting results, so no one can be certain if there is indeed such a thing as a "Parkinson's personality."

The concept of personality is somewhat fuzzy, just like descriptions of behavior in general. This is because behaviors are often indistinct. It is difficult to pin down a behavior as "abnormal" because people vary so much. It is common for close friends to agree that certain behaviors in a particular person are abnormal when they might be considered normal in others. What is considered to be a positive description by one person may be considered a negative by another.

• • • • • • • • • • • • PERSONALITY TRAITS • • • • • • • • • • •

Aloof	Friendly
Outgoing	Withdrawn
Inquisitive	Compulsive
Sensation seeking	Depressive
Obsessive	Compulsive risk taking

• •

Personality is the general term used to describe a person's demeanor and style of interacting with other people. It is a multifaceted concept and no person's personality can be captured by a single term. When therapists talk about personality *disorders*, they are describing particular areas in which the patient's skills for interacting with others are markedly abnormal. It is, however, a big leap from a personality disorder to a personality "type." A personality type is used as a general description and not as a label for something pathological. Terms such as outgoing, withdrawn, gregarious, sarcastic, social, asocial, aggressive, passive, adventurous, and timid are a partial list of personality types. Having any of these traits may be acceptable, or even good, in some situations, but too much of any of them can be abnormal. (See the table above.)

EXAMPLE

It is a good thing if your surgeon is obsessive. She will be cautious and check things. An obsessive disorder is a bad thing, because a person checks things repeatedly, to the point where it interferes with normal activities.

EXAMPLE

Being adventurous may make someone fun to be around, but being too adventurous may create dangers for others.

In the 1940s, the heyday of psychoanalysis in the United States, some physicians thought that the motor manifestations of PD actually represented physical responses to psychological stresses. Believe it or not, there are papers suggesting that PD patients' rigidity, that is, the stiffness in the muscles, was really due to a "rigid personality disorder." PD was thought to be related to "repressed emotions." PD patients were inflexible, unable to change, and, as a result, kept their muscles tight. Some PD patients had tremors because they could not psychologically deal with conflict. Conflict made them "agitated" (recall that James Parkinson himself termed this disorder, "paralysis agitans," where the term "agitans" was used as a synonym for tremor, meaning shaken up). The soft voice, the drooling, the imbalance—all were blamed on inabilities to deal with a wide spectrum of psychological issues that were transformed into physical symptoms and signs.

While these psychoanalytic notions seem quite silly to us these days, we should be careful, on the one hand, not to discard the baby with the bathwater, and, on the other hand, to always maintain a partly skeptical eye on our current research methods and beliefs. Our current understanding and treatments for PD may also look backward and perhaps even silly to our descendants.

There are many PD specialists who believe that there is such a thing as a "Parkinson's personality." Not that all PD patients are alike, but, just as not all PD patients have tremors, or speech problems, there are certain traits that seem to be more common in PD, suggesting that these traits are either part of the disease process or common responses to the various stresses and infirmities of the disease.

One problem that always crops up when PD experts think they observe patterns is that most PD specialists see in their practices a lot of PD and not too many other disorders. We sometimes believe that what we observe is unique to PD, but in fact we might find similar problems in similar frequencies in people who have nonneurological disorders such as rheumatoid arthritis, ulcerative colitis, or psoriasis. Most studies that try to determine if a personality trait is specific to PD use comparison populations. After all, lots of people suffer from depression or may be adventurous or obsessive. Just because we may see these things in PD does not mean they are not equally common in other disorders or even in the general population as well.

It is thought that Jean-Martin Charcot, the great French neurologist of the mid-1800s, was the first to think that PD patients had a particular personality. Terms such as introverted, punctual, inflexible, reliable, exacting, morally rigid, obsessive, dependent, industrious, stoic, quiet, and probably a lot more have been used.

I can state from personal experience that most of my collaborators on research projects who come from other fields comment on how much easier it is to do clinical research studies on PD patients because they are so cooperative and thoughtful. These are obviously good things, but nevertheless, it means that these researchers, with experience from other populations, do find PD patients, in some way, different.

*A*n *84-year-old man with PD spends his time at home doing nothing. I suggest a senior citizens program. I am told by the family: "He won't do it. We tried. He just refuses. He never liked to socialize."*

This is a common refrain. After a patient becomes isolated it is very difficult to overcome, especially when it occurs in a person who was never very much socially involved in the first place.

There are several issues to consider when trying to understand personality in PD. One, of course, is the tremendous variation in personality among all people, with or without disease. We all think of ourselves as unique, one of a kind, and that, while others may be somewhat like us, no other person is *exactly* like us.

So, what do we mean when we discuss personality in PD?

Question 1: Do PD patients, taken as a whole, generally share certain personality traits more than would be expected by chance alone?

If you interview a population of 100 men and women who do not have any illness, you may discover that 20 of them are gregarious and 15 of them are withdrawn; a certain percentage are adventurous;

a certain percentage are pessimistic; and so on. You then interview 100 PD patients (with similar ages) and find that 50% are pessimistic, 20% have obsessive–compulsive traits, and these numbers are very different than the comparison population. One then deduces that PD patients do have personality traits that are different from a control or comparison population. That observation will then need to be confirmed in more studies, hopefully performed in different places. This then tells us that certain personality traits are more common in PD patients. It does not tell us what the relationship is between the PD and the trait.

‘‘D*oes she think people are spying on her, or stealing? Is she paranoid?"*

"She's always been a suspicious sort of person. I don't think she's different now."

The PD medications may make people paranoid (see Chapter 9). However, some people are naturally on the "suspicious side" and are no different now than they were before the PD developed.

Question 2: Are personality trait differences in PD due to physical alterations or are they due to brain changes themselves?

Just as the loss of dopamine-containing cells in the substantia nigra may cause tremors, stiffness, rigidity, and so on, perhaps they may also cause pessimism, depression, or altered interest in sex or gambling. For instance, it may turn out that PD patients are withdrawn only if they have speech problems. Thus, being withdrawn may be purely related to a single disability and not actually be a problem intrinsic to the PD process itself. Another example may be pessimism. It may turn out that PD patients with severe disability (e.g., those who fall a lot) are pessimistic, but other PD patients are not. We would again deduce that the disability, not the disease itself, is the cause, and other people with bad knees and ankles who fall may share the same degree of pessimism. On the other hand, we may discover that PD patients with a wide variety of severe disabilities may be pessimistic and that there are no physical features we can identify to link to the pessimism. It may turn out that young patients, who one would hypothesize to be more pessimistic about their future, are no more likely to be pessimistic than 80-year-olds, or that people with minimal disabilities are just as likely to be pessimistic as wheel-chair-bound people. These findings would suggest that pessimism, or whatever traits were being examined, are not "reactive," that is, they are not the result of a particular physical problem and are more likely either related directly to what the disease does to the brain, or to what the medications do to the brain, or to some complex interaction between physical manifestations and brain pathology.

I'm not depressed. It's just that I'm frustrated. I used to be able to do everything for myself. Now I need help just to stand up. It grates on me."

This patient is not depressed. He's angry at his loss of independence. He's grieving for his lost abilities.

Question 3: Is it possible that personality alterations begin before the motor manifestations begin to alter physical behavior?

All three questions are linked.

While there have been several studies published about personality in PD, they have reached conflicting conclusions, largely because they used different research techniques, and probably because the groups of patients they studied were different. One can easily imagine that PD patients in California may be quite different from PD patients in Boston, or that Chinese PD patients in China may be very different from Americans of Chinese descent evaluated in the United States. Different results may also be expected with different comparison populations. Comparing PD patients to people with rheumatoid arthritis may produce different results than comparing them to people who had strokes or people with diabetic neuropathy.

One series of papers on this topic looked at traits thought to be "dopamine related." Dopamine is thought to be involved in the brain's reward system and is considered important in the development of addictive behavior. Dopamine is also involved in "exploratory behavior" in lab animals. Drugs that block dopamine, or surgical procedures that damage certain dopamine-containing areas of the brain, reduce lab animals' degree of exploration.

Cocaine and amphetamines—drugs of abuse—both act through increasing dopamine stimulation in the brain. Partly as a result of this observation and multiple experiments in animals, dopamine is thought to be involved in "sensation"-seeking, or novelty-seeking, behavior. Based on studies of animals and drug addicts, it therefore made sense to explore if PD patients were less likely to be novelty or sensation seekers. It also made sense to explore what effects using drugs to increase or decrease dopamine levels in the brain had on people with cocaine abuse. While dopamine-related drugs had a great effect on addicted rodents, they had little effect on addicted humans. We find that dopamine seems to be related to almost anything we study in the brain, and extrapolating behavior in experimental animals to humans is always risky.

Of course, no one would expect PD patients to bungee jump over Victoria Falls, but one could explore personality traits from before the PD developed by asking detailed questions of the patient and family members or friends about the past. One could also ask patients about interest in doing new things, seeing new movies, sampling new restaurants, meeting new people, exploring new areas, and so on.

People who smoke or drink coffee are less likely to develop PD than people who do not. This is not because cigarette smokers are more likely to die. Statistical procedures have accounted for the excess death rate among smokers. There are two differing interpretations of these results. Either there is a substance in coffee and in cigarettes that slows the onset or prevents PD from developing, or the same process that causes PD reduces the likelihood that a person will smoke or drink.

We know that dopamine is involved in addictive behaviors, and both smoking and coffee drinking may be addictive. So a dopamine deficiency, as occurs in PD, may keep someone from becoming addicted to cigarettes or coffee. This may make these substances appear as if they prevent the disease, but they obviously do not. If it was simply the lack of potential for addiction, then the idea that PD patients have different personalities because of their disease might be supported, because a tendency to addiction is a personality trait.

One study found that PD patients were less likely to have consumed two or more glasses of beer per day before their PD onset than a comparison group of the same age, with another study suggesting that even before the motor symptoms began, PD patients were more likely to have been leading a "straight and narrow" life than people without PD. The authors of one paper on this topic suggested that people who tended to have "low novelty-seeking behavior" were more likely to be "reflective, rigid, stoic, slow-tempered, frugal, persistent, and orderly."

I think I share some of these traits, and I do not currently show any symptoms of PD, but we should not believe that simply because these traits are more common in PD patients that they are in any way bad. In fact, it might be said that people with these traits are often much more likely to "succeed" in life than people who do not have these traits. Interestingly, a study that looked at personality in PD patients found only mild indications of a low novelty-seeking process, and no connection with dopamine levels in the brain—the central hypothesis of the first study. Thus, two studies had two completely different results.

Another study of premorbid (i.e., before the onset of the disease) personality traits of PD patients tried to estimate the earlier personality by asking spouses to fill out a questionnaire concerning behavior five years before the onset of the disease. Because patients had been diagnosed with PD, on average, close to six years before these interviews, spouses had to describe personality traits going back eleven or more years earlier, which was obviously a ripe source for error. Nevertheless, there were differences between the PD patients and the non-PD control group of the same age and gender distribution. PD patients were recalled as being more "generous, cautious, even-tempered, and quiet." They also were considered to be less flexible, a common theme found in many reports on PD patients. Unfortunately, the sample populations were small—only 35 in each group—and with personality traits so poorly defined, the larger the group the more likely the results are to be accurate. The authors concluded, however, that PD patients had been more introverted than average before the disease began and that this personality trait was linked to the later development of depression.

On the other hand, a study involving only 29 PD patients found no differences in personality traits between PD patients, Alzheimer's patients—both before the onset of their illnesses—and a normal comparison group. However, after the disease became evident, PD patients became more introverted, "less exploratory and curious; and less organized, goal-directed, and disciplined."

A study of twins, where only one sibling had PD, asked the subjects to fill out personality questionnaires. A group of normal volunteers of matching ages and genders was also included for comparison. The PD twins, in general, scored lower on measures of "achievement orientation" and "extraversion," but higher in "inhibitedness, somatic complaints, and emotionality." Interestingly, the twin who did not have PD often had a higher depression score than a similar individual in the healthy non-PD comparison group.

But, of course, these findings do not teach us anything about the cause of these changes. The various disabilities of PD may certainly make patients focus more on somatic complaints. The uncertain future may detract from "achievement orientation," and speech problems may account for reduced "extroversion." The increase in depressive tendencies among the non-PD twin might also simply reflect guilt or worry in the unaffected twin, which may have nothing to do with genetics. Alternatively, these finding might indicate genetic differences among the three groups.

A very interesting, although small, study looked at dependency in PD patients without dementia, compared to elderly patients without PD. They found, not surprisingly, that PD patients were more dependent and that the two major factors determining dependency were severity of motor function and depression. These factors presumably have no relationship to personality.

The questions surrounding personality in PD are both interesting and difficult. The most basic practical question is: Does it matter if PD patients have particular personality traits that are common in their disorder? On the one hand, the answer is no. What you see is what you get. A rose by any other name would smell as sweet. In other words, the personality that you or your loved one has is the personality you all have to deal with. To paraphrase ex-Secretary of Defense Donald Rumsfeld, you deal with the personality you have, not the one you wish you had.

And who is to say that's bad? And who is to say it would be different without the PD? We all have personality traits that make us different from one another, and we all respond to the tremendous amount of experiences we have had in different ways. An event may make one person more cautious and another person more adventurous. One person relishes what another avoids, just like choosing food at a restaurant. Does it matter if the PD patient's increasing caution and resistance to change is part of the disease or not?

To researcher scientists, it *does* matter. We want to know how the brain works, and one of the most important methods for figuring this out is by studying malfunctioning brains. Louis Pasteur, the great French microbiologist of the 19th century, commented that each disease was an experiment of nature. By observing these various experiments we can figure out, piece by intricate piece, how the brain works. Through these observations we sometimes can figure out how to repair the nonworking brain.

It is well known that personality *does* change in some disorders. This is an important observation, despite the fact that it seems fairly obvious. Alzheimer's patients become different people. Head-injured people may become quite different. Because personality is a characteristic of the brain, brain changes, for good or bad, may alter it. Most brain changes are, of course, bad. And, good or bad, personality changes that develop from brain disease, rather than from worldly experience, are less likely to improve things.

Since we have no methods to determine when PD actually begins in the brain, looking at premorbid symptoms is impossible. In talking about premorbid PD, we are really talking about the time before PD was recognized as being present. It is common, for example, for patients to report that they had a tremor for many years before the other symptoms of PD emerged. A decreased sense of smell, or a new problem with fatigue might have been present for several years before other problems developed. Since the connection between rapid eye movement (REM) sleep behavior disorder and PD (see Chapter 12) has been recognized, there are PD patients who report that they started having REM sleep behavior disorder 30 years before slowness or tremor developed, suggesting that PD changes had begun in the brain decades before it could be recognized. This means that personality changes could be occurring as the direct result of brain changes before PD could possibly be diagnosed. These observations make me think that PD does influence personality, but so does wealth, illness in family members, birth order, and a number of other things. I believe that PD has a modulating influence on personality, but the spectrum of personalities is so great that I think it may not be possible to point to specific traits that are "parkinsonian."

Personality determines how people diagnosed with PD deal with their illness and their lives. Some PD patients prefer to insulate themselves from the illness and act as if it wasn't there, waiting for some problem to emerge that forces them to confront their infirmity. Others seek to learn as much about PD as they can. One PD patient told me that the more he learned, the more he felt empowered, which made him feel more optimistic about his future.

Even if personality is altered by the pathology of PD itself, that is, the decline in brain cells causes the personality change, the ultimate change that we see reflects the base personality core of the individual and its blending of the PD related brain changes. However, if personality is altered by the PD changes, it suggests the possibility that some of these changes may be modifiable by drugs or stem cells. However, there is presently no treatment known to be helpful.

3

. . . .

Fatigue

People with Parkinson's disease (PD) often suffer from fatigue. About half the people with PD report that fatigue is one of their three biggest problems, and one-third report that fatigue is their single worst problem—yet our understanding of this problem is poor. In this chapter, we review fatigue in general, and specifically fatigue in PD. Some types of fatigue can be understood and treated, but some cannot. If a person with mild PD, who may look normal, says, "I'm fatigued all the time. It's my worst problem," you should know that this experience is very common. The patient is not whining.

In one major American neurology textbook, fatigue is discussed for only a few pages and is considered to be primarily psychiatric in nature. This reflects a few things. The first is that fatigue has only fairly recently been recognized as a problem in neurological disorders, after most neurologists have already completed their training.

The second is that fatigue is something doctors cannot measure. Fatigue is obviously a personal experience, which the doctor may never have had in quite the same way as the patient. Doctors are notorious for undertreating pain, even patients with pain from cancer where the disease can be clearly detected and measured. Fatigue, being a somewhat amorphous concept, is therefore even more likely than pain to be under-recognized and undertreated. And, while doctors have all suffered from pain, few have had significant problems with fatigue. If they had, they probably would not have been able to continue practicing medicine.

Third, patients with fatigue do not *suddenly* develop fatigue. Fatigue settles in gradually. It becomes an "old friend," one that the doctor may not particularly be interested in hearing about, unlike tremors or freezing or drooling, which are objective problems that can be viewed in a technical manner. The patient has sometimes already learned not to "whine" about it, as the doctor may well have given off indications that this symptom is viewed in a moral rather than scientific manner.

In addition, we have been plagued with chronic fatigue syndrome since the early 1990s, and a large percentage of these patients do suffer from major psychiatric disorders (whether these are the cause or effect is debated). The PD patients, especially the ones with minor neurological deficits but major neurological fatigue, may get tarred with the same beliefs that the doctor has about the chronic fatigue patient. Everyone feels fatigue at times. The question is, how much is normal? When do you "suck it up" and when do you bring it to the doctor's attention? The answer is very unclear.

My interest in fatigue stems from a single patient who sparked my published report linking fatigue to PD, one of the first ever published on the topic. R.O. was my age, and had very mild PD. He was working full time and doing well at work, but he would report that "the fatigue is killing me. I do my work all day but when I get home all I can do is lie on the sofa until it's time for sleep."

WHAT IS FATIGUE?

In her excellent but technical book for doctors, *Fatigue*, Lauren Krupp, MD, notes that when people are asked to describe what they mean by the word "fatigue," one gets "descriptions that range from tiredness, sleepiness, and weakness to exhaustion and languor. The truth is, fatigue can be an extremely amorphous concept, and the understanding of fatigue can vary tremendously depending on the type of patient and the background of the provider. The fact that there are so many different concepts of fatigue makes it a difficult symptom to define, assess and treat."

This certainly has been my experience. I recently interviewed two people with PD who suffered from fatigue. The two descriptions were, in my mind, very different from each other. I typed a transcription of the interviews and showed one to the other. The second patient concluded that the first patient had exactly described what he himself felt. More surprising to me was that I showed the first man four transcripts of interviews with other patients to get explanations of fatigue, and although each seemed quite different to me, this PD patient thought they were all the same—and, more importantly, all like his.

I was, and remain, quite flummoxed by this. What was I missing? I didn't know then, and I am still working on it.

There is also another definition of fatigue that is technical, related to muscle fatigue, in which individual muscles lose their strength the longer they are used. We all experience this. Lift a weight for several repetitions and after a while the muscle will become increasingly unable to lift the weight. We are not talking about individual muscle fatigue, however, when we talk about fatigue in PD. We are focusing on the general fatigue a person feels when out of energy, often due to exercise, mental or physical, or depression. A certain amount of fatigue is normal. In fact, not having fatigue may be a problem! People who are manic do not get tired. Their energy is boundless. Unfortunately, their mental powers are not able to harness this energy properly, and that sometimes gets them into trouble.

FATIGUE IN PD

Fatigue is common in PD, just as it is in many physical and mental disorders. See the following box for a partial list of disorders associated with fatigue.

•••••• DISORDERS ASSOCIATED WITH FATIGUE ••••••

Chronic fatigue syndrome
Fibromyalgia
Stroke
Radiation therapy
Starvation
Colitis or Crohn's disease
Sleep disorders
Deconditioning
Guillain–Barré syndrome
Chemotherapy
Drug effects
Endocrine disorders
Hypothyroidism

Multiple sclerosis
Head injury
Pregnancy
Infections of all types
Depression
Lou Gehrig's disease
Anemia
Heart failure
Liver diseases
Kidney diseases
Lung diseases
Systemic lupus

• •

There have been several studies of fatigue in PD. These have had relatively consistent results. About half of people with PD rate fatigue as one of the worst three symptoms of PD, including the typical motor aspects of PD such as tremor, slowness, gait dysfunction, and so on. About one-third of PD patients rate fatigue as their single worst symptom. In a drug study of newly diagnosed, very mildly affected PD patients, one-third considered fatigue as a significant problem.

PD patients report their fatigue as being different from the fatigue they experienced prior to the onset of the disease, although in what ways it is different has often not been reported. As with depression in PD, fatigue is a problem that overlaps with other symptoms to such a degree that it is hard to study in isolation. Even our language contributes to the difficulty. We describe being "tired" as feeling physically fatigued, but we also use the term at the end of the day, particularly after a poor night's sleep, to say we are "tired" and need to sleep. We also say we need to "rest," which is an ambiguous term that can be used to mean resting from an exertion by sitting or lying down, as well as napping to catch up with sleep deprivation.

TYPES OF FATIGUE

We sometimes think of two major types of fatigue, physical and mental. Mental fatigue refers to the feeling people develop after studying or working very hard. A person who spends weeks preparing a law case, a business proposal, or a school report may develop mental fatigue. Bertrand Russell, the British philosopher who spent several years working closely with another philosopher to write a massive mathematics and logic text laying the foundation for all of mathematics, was so drained from the experience that he gave up all such similar pursuits for the rest of his life.

In ordinary life, we do not have such experiences, but we certainly do tire from reading difficult books, filling out our income taxes, completing our children's college applications, and myriad other things that demand a lot of time and intense concentration. We reach a point where we cannot concentrate any longer and need a rest. We generally think of this as intellectual fatigue, one form of mental fatigue.

Perhaps more common for most adults is emotional fatigue. We become highly involved in some activity that demands a degree of emotional involvement that is difficult to sustain; for example, a child's marriage, a grandchild's school activities, a spouse's business ventures, our friendships, and marriages. These are not physically demanding, but the emotional requirements may produce the same sense of fatigue and are equally as universal a phenomenon.

The sense of fatigue in patients with PD is generally a physical sensation, but, to be honest, and I hope you do not find this to be too surprising, I am not completely certain about this. I am considered to be an expert in the field, having published some research papers. But this is a field in its infancy. In fact, the first two papers addressing the topic of fatigue in PD were published in 1992, each independent of the other. Consider this in context: One of the most common and bothersome aspects of PD was not recognized as even being a problem until 175 years after James Parkinson published his monograph! (This always makes me worry about the things I may be missing each day.)

So then, what exactly is fatigue? I used to think I knew it when I felt it, but the more I learn the less I think I know. I have interviewed my PD patients who claim to feel fatigue, to try to get a better understanding of it. But the more people I interview, the more I sometimes think that I will never "understand" it.

Interview

Here is an interview with a 79-year-old woman with a 13-year history of PD and severe dyskinesias (the involuntary movements caused by long use of L-Dopa).

Q: You said that the dyskinesias make you feel tired.
A: Yes. Exhausted.

Q: And you told me that this fatigue—you used the word fatigue—is different from feeling sleepy. Is that correct?
A: Yes.

Q: Can you describe the difference?
A: When I'm sleepy, I'm sleepy. With the dyskinesias, I'm just tired.

Q: We talked before about what the tiredness felt like when you exercised before you had Parkinson's.
A: Exercising made me feel regenerated and rejuvenated. I felt good after I exercised, even though I was tired. But now I don't feel good. I'm just plain tired.

Q: Are you achy?
A: Sometimes. My legs and my back ache.

Q: When is the fatigue the worst?
A: After a couple of hours of this.

Q: You told me that you feel restless at times.

A: Yes. And the fatigue is worse after I feel this restlessness.

Q: You mentioned that you had always had a problem with fatigue even before the Parkinson's, even though you worked full-time and had two kids. How was that fatigue different from the fatigue that you feel now?

A: I think it was because, back then I was busy and tired. Now I'm not as busy, but I get tired easier.

Q: So you think you have more time to think about it?

A: Probably.

Q: Do you nap at all during the day?

A: I lie down and rest for about an hour each day.

Q: Do you sleep during that hour?

A: Sometimes, but it is only for 10 or 15 minutes.

Q: Does sleeping make you feel refreshed?

A: Not always.

Q: Does sleeping improve your tiredness?

A: Not always. Sometimes I get up and feel just as tired as before I slept.

Q: Now, again, I'm trying to understand the difference between the fatigue that you feel and the fatigue that I feel myself if I walk 10 miles. Is your fatigue associated with some type of tension?

A: Yes, I think so. When I start, right now, with my medication wearing off and I'm starting this I'm fine, I'm not as tired. But when the dyskinesias start, I'm exhausted.

Q: So the dyskinesias make you feel tired to the point of being exhausted?

A: Yes.

Q: If you were to rate your problems with Parkinson's, would fatigue be in the top three?
A: Probably.

Q: Do you feel tired for more than half the day?
A: Yes.

Q: Do you feel tired for three-fourths of the day?
A: Yes.

Q: And yet you lead a pretty active life.
A: Well, I made up my mind that I wasn't going to just sit around doing nothing. I was going to try to keep busy and do things. The only thing I'm not doing is driving.

Q: You look pretty restless right now. Are you?
A: Yes.

Q: And are you feeling fatigued right now?
A: No.

Q: So, sometimes you can be restless and have dyskinesias and not feel fatigue. But other times you do feel fatigued.
A: After a couple of hours of the dyskinesias, then I'm tired.

Q: Are there any tricks you have for dealing with fatigue?
A: No.

Q: Here's an interesting question. If we stopped your medicine for a day or two, and your dyskinesias went away completely but you started to shake and maybe you were stooped or you had more trouble walking, what do you think would happen to your fatigue? Would it be better, worse, or the same?
A: Probably worse.

Q: So you think that even though the dyskinesias make you feel fatigued, you think that being unmedicated, stiff, and slow would make you feel more fatigued?

A: Yes, because then I would feel as though I couldn't do anything. Exercising has always helped, and I enjoy exercising.

Q: You told me that you haven't been exercising this winter.

A: Well, the last couple of weeks. I was doing exercises as therapy.

Q: And that helped your fatigue?

A: Yes.

Q: So, if we had you exercise more, your fatigue would improve?

A: Yes, I think so.

There are a number of interesting points here. For one thing, exercise makes this PD patient feel better. This is a much different phenomenon from what occurs in fatigued normal people. When I'm tired, I don't want to do more exercise, and when I'm forced to do more, then I get more fatigued. If I get tired after jogging five miles, the notion that I'll feel *less* fatigued if I jog another mile does not seem to make sense. Yet, this fatigued patient with PD reports just this phenomenon.

In addition, she has an easy-to-understand problem that contributes to her fatigue—her dyskinesias. If you have ever watched someone with severe dyskinesias, it is hard to keep from jumping out of your own skin. The poor patient is writhing and jerking nonstop, sometimes even building up a sweat. It is easy to understand why these patients are fatigued from their excessive, constant exercising, even when not meaning to. On very rare occasions, PD patients have to dramatically reduce their medications to avoid having a heart attack, because their medication-induced movements produce so much exercise, hence a strain on the heart. Yet this patient states that if we stopped her medications, she would feel even greater fatigue, "because then I would feel as though I couldn't do anything."

Another fascinating aspect of this patient's story is the report that despite feeling tired most of the day, every day, she nevertheless leads an active lifestyle.

Here is an interview with a man who developed PD at age 44, now 57.

Q: Fatigue was your biggest problem back in the early days.
A: It was a very large problem because it took so much away from my day and also my family's day. Even today, my wife knows when I've been taking my medicine [a stimulant] to give me more energy or not.

Q: Can you describe what you mean when you use the word "fatigue"?
A: There are two things. One is that I always want to lie down. I never feel energetic. I never feel as if I want to run around the house or go outdoors and enjoy things. I feel as though I am very tired.

Q: When you say you are tired or fatigued, can you distinguish that feeling from feeling sleepy?
A: Yes, I think I can. It is more that I lack the enthusiasm to get up and get going to do stuff. It is not as if I want to go to sleep, like at night. I am just totally run down. That's a better description.

Q: Do you nap during the day?
A: Very seldom.

Q: If you do nap, does that give you more energy?
A: No. Because I don't think it is good rest that I get. I believe that over the years I've become more a person set in my ways,

where a nap doesn't fit into my routine. My routine is that I go to bed at night and get up in the morning and I'm awake for the whole day.

Q: And you sleep fairly well at night?
A: I do. It is a short sleep, maybe six hours or so. But it is a very sound sleep.

Q: So you are not bothered by excess sleepiness during the day?
A: Not since I've been put on the stimulant medication.

The problem with understanding fatigue is that it means different things to different people, and it is associated with so many different conditions. In the interviews above we learned that exercise, which is usually the last thing most fatigued people want to do, makes an elderly woman with PD feel more energetic! Yet, the middle-aged man, who has had PD just as long, cannot bring himself to exercise and has a hard time starting any activities at all. The first patient is fatigued by her dyskinesias. They are so prominent that it is hard to understand how she even takes in enough calories to keep up with her energy needs. Yet exercise makes her feel better. Other patients report that once they start an activity it is hard to continue because every activity is an effort.

We studied energy expenditure in PD patients with fatigue. First, we conducted an experiment to measure how much energy it took just to breathe. PD patients use more energy to breathe than people without PD. This makes sense because PD affects the muscles in the chest and the diaphragm. This makes the breathing activity less efficient. I thought that this may be one reason PD patients are more likely to be fatigued. They start off "wasting" energy. Every motor act is inefficient compared to someone without PD. PD patients can do chores that look easy, but those chores may seem to the patient like two or three times as much work because of their muscular inefficiency.

We learned from our measurements that there were no differences. All PD patients were less efficient than normal people, but exercise efficiency did not distinguish the fatigued and nonfatigued PD patients. We found that fatigued PD patients were more depressed, in general, than nonfatigued patients, but there were still many PD patients who were not depressed despite being fatigued.

As you might expect from the results of this experiment, fatigue was unrelated to the severity of the PD. In fact, in a follow-up study, we found that most fatigued patients remained fatigued and that very few patients became fatigued if they weren't already fatigued. This means that we found that fatigue establishes itself early in the course of the PD and tends to remain a problem. Unfortunately, it also got worse with time.

Another report, from Europe, obtained somewhat different results. While a lot of their fatigued patients did remain fatigued over a few years, some stopped being fatigued, and patients who had had the disease for a few years developed fatigue. At this time we don't know which is true, and it doesn't matter for any individual patient. If they're fatigued, they're fatigued. However, the observation that some people develop fatigue and then recover suggests that at least some of the fatigued patients are treatable.

It also suggests that there are probably different types of fatigue. I have been impressed that patients whose PD is very minor may complain of severe fatigue, while other patients, who are extremely slow and tremor a lot, have very little fatigue. I wonder sometimes if part of the problem is expectation. Many fatigued PD patients may expect so much from themselves that they have difficulty adjusting to the difference between what they expect and what they can do. However, even if this is correct, this theory would only explain a small part of the problem.

In a classic report on PD from 1967, Hoehn and Yahr reported that 2% of their PD patients listed fatigue as their principal reason for seeing a neurologist. Most of their patients sought consultation for slowness, tremor, or gait problems. Thus, on the one hand, 2% is a small number; on the other hand, 2% of their patients did seek help because unexplained fatigue was their major problem. Most likely these patients had PD without tremor, and the other aspects of PD were not perceived as problems.

Many people with fatigue will "rest" to overcome it. When they "rest" they may or may not fall asleep. Whether they sleep or not, they may feel refreshed for a while after the rest but then become fatigued again. It is unclear, often to the patient herself, whether the sleeping was important or just lying down and relaxing was the important part. Because sleep problems are so common in PD, it is always a consideration in the understanding of fatigue. Many of the sleep problems aren't even perceived by the patient or the family.

The relationship between depression and fatigue is probably more complex. It is one of those chicken-and-egg questions. How much does depression make you fatigued or how much does fatigue make you depressed? People who are depressed feel run down and tired all the time. Everything is an effort. When they start a project, they have difficulty completing it because of being so tired. The effort is so great that there is little enjoyment in whatever activity is taking place. "Yes, I'd like to go to the movie, but I really don't feel up to it. I think I'll stay home." "I need to mow the lawn, but I just don't have the energy." "Exercise would make me feel better, but I can't get myself to start." "I don't enjoy taking walks anymore because I feel so tired."

FATIGUE AND DEPRESSION

This association is a far more difficult theoretical problem to unravel than the association of fatigue with sleep. On the positive side, however, it is much easier to treat practically. If I cannot tell if a patient's fatigue is due to depression, I treat the depression. If the depression improves and the fatigue resolves, then the problem is solved. If the mood and other symptoms of depression improve but the fatigue does not, then there are two separate problems. Of course, we are often left with the difficult issue of the patient who does not improve in any way after taking the antidepressant. In this case, are we dealing with a drug failure, or does the patient not suffer from depression? The problem looks like this. The patient feels fatigued.

He doesn't enjoy things anymore, "because they are too hard to do. I just don't have the energy." His sleep habits have deteriorated because he sits around and can't keep from napping on and off all day. He feels frustrated, angry, irritable, and withdraws from the world. Naturally, his mood is not so hot. So, is he depressed or is he simply frustrated by the limitations of his fatigue?

One of the central features of depression is fatigue. As far as we know now, there are no particular differences between the fatigue of depression and the fatigue of PD. But what might some differences be? Perhaps their daily cycles may be different. It is easy to imagine that a PD patient may become more fatigued as the day progresses and he "uses up" his energy. On the other hand, one can imagine that a depressed patient may awaken in the morning and face another 16 hours of unrelenting misery, perhaps feeling less and less burdened as the day progresses and bedtime draws closer. A depressed patient may be more likely to do things if left alone, whereas a PD patient may be more likely to do things under social pressure.

Perhaps there are also other ways to distinguish the fatigue symptoms, but so far no one knows how to do this. Maybe there are no differences. One study successfully treated fatigue in non-PD patients that remained after other symptoms of depression improved with an antidepressant. This suggests that fatigue is a symptom related to, but distinct from, depression.

FATIGUE VERSUS APATHY

PD patients may say, "I'm too tired," when they want to avoid doing something. Apathetic patients don't care about too much. They are most comfortable not dealing with the world, sitting in their own microcosms. Like people in a rut, they require what for them is a large expenditure of energy to do anything out of the ordinary. This approach to chores, socializing, activities of all sorts looks a lot like "lacking energy," which is one way of describing fatigue. When asked why they don't leave the house or socialize in any way, they may say that it's "too hard." Every activity that is out of the usual routine becomes enormously difficult, and fatigue is one potential explanation for this, just as apathy may be as well. The major difference between apathy and fatigue, I believe, is that the fatigued patient is upset or frustrated by this, whereas the apathetic patient doesn't care and isn't particularly interested in finding treatment for the fatigue.

Motivation and fatigue are closely related, as are motivation and apathy.

FATIGUE AND EXERCISE

Because fatigue in PD is not fully understood, one can try to extrapolate from other conditions that are associated with fatigue. Regular exercise has been shown to reduce fatigue in cancer patients undergoing various kinds of therapy. Some PD patients, as in the example above, report that exercise actually reduces the fatigue, although this certainly is not a universal observation. Many PD patients complain that exercise makes their fatigue much worse, while many others say they would love to exercise but cannot because they are too fatigued to begin the process. For some people, fatigue seems to have a large component of impaired motivation. "The mind is willing but the flesh is weak." The patient may very much like to exercise but simply lacks the energy to get moving. How many of us plan to exercise regularly, lose weight, stop smoking, and so on but cannot quite get going to actually do it?

A study published in 2005 reported that in a large group of health professionals followed for many years, vigorous physical activity was associated with a lower risk of developing PD in men (but not also in women, for unknown reasons). They also reported that exercise fell off in men starting twelve years before PD was diagnosed and two to four years before diagnosis in women. Other studies of large groups have shown that people who are more physically active are less likely to develop fatigue, regardless of developing PD or any other particular illness.

Several studies have demonstrated that PD patients who exercise have improved physical function, gait, and quality of life. None of these studies have looked specifically at fatigue, but exercise in other disorders plus the known association between quality of life and fatigue suggest that exercise most likely reduces fatigue.

In a variety of medical disorders, including congestive heart failure, depression, diabetes, hypertension, and coronary artery disease, the time spent exercising predicted the level of vitality two years later. It is hard to believe that this would not apply to PD as well.

TREATING FATIGUE

There is no known treatment for fatigue in PD. Obviously the first thing to do is to carefully figure out what the patient means by the term. How much does sleep disturbance contribute? How much may be due to depression? How much may be apathy or frustration? How much exercise does the person do? How much is an excuse to avoid embarrassment in social interactions? Clearly, all of these factors need to be addressed as well as they can be. What is left is what I label as fatigue.

My own approach to treating fatigue is to try the selective serotonin reuptake inhibitor antidepressants (Prozac, Zoloft, Paxil, Lexapro, Celexa, etc.) that are not sedating and may be "activating" according to psychiatrists, once we have improved sleep as much as possible. Sometimes I try modafinil (Provigil) to keep the patient awake during the day if excessive daytime sleepiness is a problem. I also encourage exercise, even if it is only five minutes of walking at a time. The goal then becomes to walk five minutes at a time more than once each day, then to increase the time by one minute or more each week, eventually getting to a thirty-minute walk each day.

If walking fails, I try stimulant medication, using drugs such as methamphetamine, methylphenidate, and similar drugs. These drugs are used in hyperactive children to slow them down. They are also "uppers" used by truck drivers to keep from falling asleep, college kids to cram overnight, overweight people to lose weight, and drug addicts. These drugs are not safe for everyone. As of the end of 2012, only a single study has reported successful treatment of fatigue in PD. The researchers used low-dose methylphenidate (Ritalin), a drug used primarily to treat children with attention deficit disorder. Nonstimulant drugs that prevent sleepiness, such as modafinil (Provigil) and armodafinil (Nuvigil), have not been helpful in treating fatigue in PD.

Amphetamine was tested as a treatment for PD in the 1970s and was found to not be helpful, although not harmful. The major contraindication for using stimulants in PD patients is heart disease, both ischemia (coronary artery disease, angina, history of heart attack) and arrhythmia. Any patient with a history of drug abuse also should probably not take a stimulant. With my own patients, I believe that stimulants are sometimes helpful, but this could be a placebo effect. I do not think my patients are getting "high," although this could be hidden from me, or the medication may simply be keeping the patients more alert and awake. They may be worth trying if all else fails, until we in the PD research community get around to studying this properly.

INTERESTING ASPECTS OF FATIGUE

Some forms of fatigue appear to be immune system related. The interferons, drugs that work on the immune system, universally produce prominent fatigue. The autoimmune diseases—disorders in which the body attacks itself, such as lupus erythematosis or rheumatoid arthritis—are highly associated with fatigue. Radiation therapy induces fatigue, even though many cancers themselves do not! The time course of the fatigue is predictable, and while the feeling of fatigue is predictable, the physiology of the fatigue remains unknown. A 2012 study of patients who had suffered minor strokes found that fatigue was a very common new problem after the stroke. The researchers found that fatigue correlated to some degree with depression but did not correlate with the amount of dysfunction caused by the stroke and did not correlate with any particular part of the brain that was affected by the stroke. In other words, there is no "fatigue" center in the brain.

One fascinating observation is that fatigue is more prominent in patients who have made a good recovery from Guillain–Barré syndrome, a disorder of the peripheral nerves causing weakness and numbness, than those who have made a poor recovery. In other words the stronger patients felt more fatigued than the weaker!

There have been no plausible theories for what causes fatigue. My own view is that there are many possible explanations, even within the same disorder. Some degree of fatigue is due to depression; some is due to a discrepancy between what a person feels he should be able to do and what he actually can do; some is likely due to hormonal or chemical changes induced by the disease.

4

. . . .

Apathy

Many Parkinson's disease (PD) patients lose some of their motivation as they discover routine tasks to become increasingly challenging. They often begin to lose interest in things going on around them, as well as in their long-standing hobbies and pleasures. While some of these changes may be the result of motor function and frustration, we believe that much of it is due to changes in regions of the brain that control motivation and reward. This "apathy" rarely bothers the patient. The patient "doesn't care." It bothers family and friends, though, because it seems to them that the PD patient is "giving in" to the disease, succumbing in spirit. The patient generally is psychologically removed and insulated from the distress. It is presently unknown if this apathy can be treated.

WHAT IS APATHY?

One of the most difficult problems for family members of patients with PD is apathy. Apathy is defined in one psychiatry text as a "dulled emotional tone associated with detachment or indifference." In general parlance, apathy means without feeling.

We often use the term "apathetic" to describe someone who shows no emotional responses to anything. "He doesn't care" is synonymous with "he's apathetic." We usually think of being apathetic applying to specific targets. "She doesn't care about sports." "He's not interested in poetry." "She doesn't care about money." It is normal to have areas of interest and areas of disinterest. In PD, as part of the illness, many patients increasingly stop caring about things going on around them, even things that used to interest them and that theoretically should still interest them. This is a very challenging clinical problem because it is not well understood, often not recognized, and is usually distressing to the family. Additionally, apathy may be difficult to distinguish from depression, and it always causes more problems for the caregivers and family than for the patient.

Apathy describes a collection of behavioral changes that includes lessened interest in events, reduced spontaneous interactions with others or with pets, decreased concern or seeming indifference to friends and family, muted emotional tone, loss of interest in hobbies, loss of enjoyment as well as loss of distress at hearing bad news, and loss of motivation.

Richard Brown, a prominent neuropsychologist, noted that, "Apathy has a direct impact on the overall level of handicap." Because apathetic patients are not invested in getting better, they do not participate in activities that help maintain function. Apathy in a patient increases the caregiver's burden and, perhaps most importantly, decreases the feeling of reward the caregiver experiences. It has clear implications for long-term treatment and therefore outcome, and both of these are not good. On the other hand, one must also see the protective effect that apathy has on the patient himself. He cares less, hence grieves and suffers less for the losses caused by the PD.

A *75-year-old woman with a 20-year history of PD has been suffering from dementia for about five years. She follows a regular routine of senior daycare five days each week. She lives with her daughter, who is an elementary school teacher. For about two years the patient had been suffering from psychotic symptoms such as hallucinations and delusions, and she has also been very anxious.*

At a recent visit, the daughter reported that her mother has been increasingly "tranquil." "She's in a good place now most of the time. She seems comfortable, with only occasional problems with anxiety."

The tranquility described was really apathy. The patient wasn't happy or sad or nervous or concerned about anything. She simply floated on a calm emotional sea. To the daughter this was a good thing. Her mother was not suffering anymore.

In psychiatric parlance apathy is a "negative symptom." It is the absence of something normal. Apathetic patients, when asked what they are thinking about will often answer, "Nothing." They think and feel less than they had before, and as the condition worsens they think and feel less and less.

Apathy reportedly affects about 40% to 45% of patients with PD, but I believe this is an overestimate. Apathy is often mistaken for a symptom of depression, malaise from illness, sleepiness, overmedication, or pain. For example, most of us would not classify someone as apathetic if they were in pain and focused only on the pain, ignoring the rest of the world.

WITH WHAT IS APATHY CONFUSED?

Many depressed people "don't care," and therefore they seem apathetic. As Dr. Brown commented, "The challenge for studies of depression in PD ... is to distinguish patients with primary apathy versus apathy that is a feature of a depressive disturbance." This problem cuts both ways, with apathetic patients diagnosed with depression and vice versa. Apathy, like depression, is also confused with fatigue and may be a response to repeated frustrations.

The central differences between apathy and depression include irritability, reduced effort, sadness, sleep disturbances, and anxiety. Apathetic people don't have these problems, whereas depressed people often do.

The main similarities between apathy and depression are anhedonia (absence of enjoyment), loss of motivation, and lack of interest.

IS APATHY A PROBLEM?

Apathy is a significant problem in one way, but not necessarily in others. When I think a patient is apathetic, I always point out to the family that the patient is not suffering, only they are. When the patient is apathetic, he doesn't care. He doesn't care if the TV is on one station or another, or he may not care if it isn't even on at all. He doesn't care that he doesn't care. The family will say that the patient spends the whole day sitting in the chair, looking out the window or looking at the TV, falling asleep. He doesn't ask for food, although he'll eat when given. The spouse is understandably upset and concerned. It is helpful, I believe, to counsel the family that the only one *not* suffering is the patient. He, of course, doesn't care.

However, just as this revised edition was going to press, Nathanial Stevens emailed me about his experience with apathy and I find his insight valuable. He does not suffer from depression, memory impairment, or other behavioral problems.

Though I agree that it is harder on my family, I have to disagree about the patient's suffering. You see, I do have apathy and on an emotional level everything is dulled (the best way I can think to describe it). My intellect, however, is functioning just fine. On an intellectual level I know that my apathy is painful for my wife in particular. This causes me pain on some level, though not emotionally per se. Therefore I won't allow myself to succumb to it completely. I have been using that one still very high functioning part of my brain, my intellect, to try to overcome the apathy. It's not easy, and it's not a fight I always win, but it works much of the time.

One of the near-universal responses I hear when I ask a family if the patient enjoys anything is the answer "the grandchildren" or "the children."

However, on interviewing the patient and family, it becomes clear that while the patient does enjoy these visits, the enjoyment is very short-lived, and in the case of very active younger children, the enjoyment is soon counterbalanced by the uncomfortable excess activity. Like everything else, apathy in PD is not an "all-or-none" phenomenon. It develops slowly, with a continual decline in the level of interest and level of enjoyment. Just as no one can identify one particular date when bradykinesia began, although they can sometimes tell the date when it was first noticed, no one can exactly point out when apathy first set in. The first thing that is usually lost is socializing, "because it's hard." Then it becomes evident that it is not just the effort, physical or mental, but it is also the upset in the routine, and then the lack of reward to compensate for the upset routine.

While apathy may not bother the patient very much, it still has major implications for the patient and the family. It has a significant deleterious effect on the caregiver as well as the patient. It is a well-established fact that in all diseases, those with a positive attitude, in general, do better in every measure of health and life satisfaction than those who do not. While apathetic patients are not necessarily pessimistic, they are not optimistic either. The attitude is hard on the caregivers and family because their extra efforts to do something particularly nice, and even their daily efforts, no matter how extraordinary, are not rewarded with the depth of gratitude appropriate to the efforts and sacrifice.

Apathy is more common in patients who are demented, but not all apathetic patients are demented. The onset of apathy begins with emotional withdrawal, an easy to understand response to the progressively impairing symptoms of PD. If it is difficult being understood, it is natural to participate less in conversations. The less one interacts socially, whether due to poor articulation, tremor, drooling or anything else, the easier it becomes to grow increasingly isolated. The more isolated one becomes the more one builds up a protective attitude of not caring. The more "not caring" someone becomes, the less interested they become in their interactions, and then, of course, the more apathetic they feel toward these activities. It is a vicious cycle.

Not caring can be very protective. As one becomes increasingly unable to perform certain activities, the starker the effects of the

PD become. To not care about these changes is therefore extremely helpful in warding off the possible depression—inducing feelings of decline. Not caring versus feeling "disgusted" with oneself or "frustrated" may be easier on the psyche. It can be impossible to determine at times whether the lack of caring, that is, apathy, is due to frustration or depression, that is, whether it is a reaction to the motor disability or simply part of the disease process.

In the few studies of apathy in PD, however, it was not found to correlate with disease severity, as measured by motor function or by duration of the disease. A British study found that apathy did correlate with cognitive dysfunction but that it was not related to physical impairment, depression, or anxiety. Thus, attempts to treat apathy by treating depression are not likely to be very helpful.

A British study that compared PD patients with equally impaired osteoarthritis (OA) patients found apathy to be much more common in PD. The arthritics were chosen as the comparison (control) group because they were roughly the same age and had similar degrees of disability from an equally incurable disorder. Of course, OA is different from PD. It doesn't affect the voice. It doesn't slow down the thinking. It doesn't cause drooling or shaking, and almost every older person has some degree of arthritis, so the disability is well understood by almost everyone.

One hypothesis they tested was whether the PD patients may have developed "premature social aging" as a result of their disabilities. In other words, did they spend more time in solitary activities such as watching TV, looking out the window, reading the newspaper, and generally avoiding social contact simply because it was difficult to overcome the obstacles to doing something social? "The osteoarthritis sample, despite their disability, showed no evidence of apathy." This pointed to apathy being part of the PD (or the PD medications), but not just due to physical disabilities. There was no difference between PD patients who had tremors and those who did not. Apathy did not correlate with disease duration or motor disability. While there was a correlation between apathy and cognitive function, few patients were actually demented.

Another result was the lack of connection between personality and apathy. Some had hypothesized that certain personality traits, notably "novelty-seeking behavior," would be negatively correlated with apathy, that is, people whose native personality thrived on doing unusual things would be less likely to lose interest in activities. But this turned out to be incorrect.

The most important observation in this study was that patients with high levels of apathy also had the poorest executive function, one of the measures of problem solving and memory capabilities. Yet, these patients were not demented. They had no memory problems and functioned normally in social settings and at their jobs. The authors thought that apathy might "mark a subtype of PD."

Interview

A 78-year-old man with PD for six years has been increasingly incapacitated by his gait and balance problems. When asked about his lifestyle, he reports that it is "OK." When asked about his mood, he responds that it too is "OK."

Q: What do you do for fun?
A: Not much.

Q: Does it bother you?
A: No.

Q: Do you watch TV much?
A: The TV is on most of the time.

Q: What do you watch?
A: The History Channel or sports.

Q: Do you visit friends?
A: No, it's too difficult.

Q: Do they visit you?
A: They used to, but they stopped.

Q: Does that bother you?
A: Not really.

The patient's wife and children report that he spends the whole day watching the TV and falling asleep. He never complains about being bored but appears to have an interest in nothing. The only time he perks up is when the grandchildren visit, but this happiness lasts only for 15 minutes, then he starts becoming anxious because the activity level is too high and overwhelms him.

This is a very common scenario. On the one hand, the apathetic attitude is devastating to the family, who sees themselves robbed of a formerly vital and vibrant, entertaining man, but on the other hand, it is somewhat protective in that the patient no longer worries about himself or feels frustrated by his inability to do the things that had been second nature to him and a great source of enjoyment.

A 60-year-old woman has lost interest in her friends and relatives. She had been very social, and involved in her grandchildren and her church. Her PD is mild, and should not really interfere with her activities, although her tremor is a major cosmetic problem. It doesn't really interfere with her ability to perform her activities, but she has been so self-conscious that she has withdrawn from many public activities because people stare at her. She denies feeling sad, but admits to a lack of enjoyment. She feels fatigued, but ascribes this to poor sleeping at night, due to anxieties over how much of a burden she's becoming to her children who have their small children to care for. Her weight is down, which she thinks is due to the slowed eating from her PD.

The clinical question in this vignette is whether the patient is depressed, apathetic without depression, excessively fatigued, or excessively sleepy. There is so much overlap among these symptoms that even an experienced PD specialist in psychiatry or neurology may not know how to classify the problem. In fact, the patient has all of the problems. The real issue is which is the "main" problem. Depression may cause all these symptoms, as may fatigue, anxiety, and sleep dysfunction.

In approaching such a patient, the first thing to realize is that treating the motor dysfunction, in this case the tremor, is probably not going to accomplish much. The tremor does not interfere with function, and although it causes distress, tremor always surfaces when the patient is stressed, so no medication is going to prevent that. Therefore, the focus must be on what is treatable.

Probably the easiest problems to approach are those related to sleep and anxiety, which are interrelated, and the fatigue or possible depression. It is important to keep in mind that not all depressed patients report sadness. There are forms of depression in which the patient does not feel "blue" or "down," and, in addition, there are patients who are reluctant to report feeling sad. I might therefore treat the patient with an antidepressant that has antianxiety properties, or I might use a sleep medication at night, most of which also are antianxiety medications. Another approach might be to send the patient to a sleep laboratory to check for sleep problems, but I think that would probably not alter the approach to treatment.

A *73-year-old man falls asleep frequently and does not seem to care. His family finds that he is not interested in anything. He attends family get-togethers and falls asleep before too long. He goes to his grandchildren's little league and soccer games and falls asleep. He is not embarrassed. He merely reports that, "I'm tired a lot." He has severe PD and is generally transported in a wheelchair. He is mildly demented, confusing some of his grandchildren from time to time, but never seems sad or anxious. He sleeps 12 hours each night and naps after breakfast. He snores mightily.*

This patient probably suffers from sleep apnea and clearly has a sleep disorder. Some of his dementia may, in fact, be sleep related, and his lack of interest in anything also may be largely sleep driven, or at least exacerbated by his constant sleepiness. It is likely that this patient's life could be improved considerably if the sleep apnea could be treated. Unfortunately, not too many PD patients are able to tolerate the various mechanical treatments for sleep apnea. Medications have not been helpful so far.

A very interesting although preliminary study that I helped design involved evaluating men with PD for apathy and then comparing their apathy scores to their level of testosterone. We conducted the study because other researchers had reported that PD males who suffered from depression yet failed to respond to antidepressant medications often had low testosterone levels. This observation, not yet confirmed, suggested the possibility that some behavior problems in PD might be partly or completely related to other, medical—in this case endocrine—disorders. We know that other endocrine disorders, such as low thyroid hormone levels, are associated with depression, fatigue, and apathy. We also know that low testosterone, which is thought to be a rare problem in men, is associated with behavioral changes, such as diminished aggressiveness, decreased energy, and fatigue. We do not know how often men with PD have low testosterone levels.

My study revealed that it was surprisingly common. This does not mean that low testosterone is the cause of the apathy. In depressed patients, giving them testosterone does not help their depression. It is quite possible that the apathy caused the low testosterone. Perhaps men who were not interested in almost anything were not interested in sexual things, which then reduced the levels of testosterone. Or perhaps there is some intermediary condition that caused both the low testosterone and the apathy.

TREATMENT

There is no known treatment for apathy. Theories abound on which neurotransmitter systems are involved, and although a popular theory implies that dopamine is involved, there is a lot of evidence that L-Dopa and the dopamine agonists only have a minimal effect on this problem in PD.

When apathy is believed to be related to depression or sleep disorders, these problems should be treated. Hopefully, the apathy will then improve. If there is a medical reason for the apathy such as low hormone levels, abnormal kidney function, or abnormal liver function, then the medical reason needs to be addressed first.

One possibility to consider is that apathy is a "protective" response and not "organic." By "organic" we mean that it is part of the illness, a direct result of losing neurons or neurotransmitters in crucial brain locations. By "protective" or "psychodynamic," we mean that there may be a psychological reason, although not conscious to the patient. But patients may be so aware of their dependent condition, of their burden on others, that they may slowly adapt a mental attitude of indifference.

They are tired of constantly apologizing for all the work they have caused. They are tired of feeling guilty for wetting the bed because they cannot roll over and get out of bed under their own steam. They are tired of feeling guilty for keeping spouses from enjoying themselves, for suffering a poorer standard of living, for not having vacations planned, or retirement, and a host of other things. Instead of feeling depressed, irritable, and angry, some people may become introverted and apathetic. It is likely that this is a form of depression and may well respond to antidepressants.

One approach to treating apathy advocated by some psychiatrists is the use of dopamine agonists. These are pramipexole, ropinerole, pergolide, bromocriptine, and cabergoline. While these are fine to use, it is important to keep in mind the fact that there is no data to support their use for this problem. That is, they may *theoretically* work, but, more importantly, they have the potential for mental side effects.

My own approach, which I think is probably the most common, is to try one or two antidepressants, on the assumptions that the drugs are generally well tolerated, and there is always the possibility that the apathy represents a symptom of depression.

It is very clear that this is a topic that needs much more research attention.

5

. . . .

Depression

Depression is common in Parkinson's disease (PD), but is difficult to define. Many of the signs we use to recognize depression in normal people are part of the motor problems in PD and have nothing to do with mood. This problem has resulted in markedly varying estimates of how common depression is in PD. Complicating this further is the small number of studies of treating depression. After many years where neurologists and psychiatrists have been telling their colleagues to be sensitive to recognize depression, but had no evidence to prove that treatment worked, we now have such evidence.

THE NATURE OF DEPRESSION IN PD

"Wouldn't *you* be depressed if you had a progressive, incurable, and often disabling disease?" This question is perhaps the fundamental base on which the whole field of neuropsychiatry is founded. Do PD patients become depressed because of the physical challenges of their illness, that is, is the depression due to the death of certain particular brain cells, or do PD patients become depressed because of the psychological challenges of their illness, that is, is the depression due to their disabilities and uncertain future?

The answer is "Yes." What I mean is that this theoretically interesting question actually has little meaning to a person with PD. It has become very clear, but only in recent years, that depression is undoubtedly due to both causes.

"Yeah, I feel depressed. I'm really ticked off. I can't drive my car anymore because of the PD. I can't eat my favorite dessert since I developed diabetes. My doctor told me to lay off the salty food because of my blood pressure. I started falling so I can't walk my dog anymore. These 'golden years' aren't what they're cracked up to be."

While this patient may be depressed, at this point he is more angry from frustration than he is depressed. This is not the sort of problem that is likely to benefit from an antidepressant medication and probably needs some "talk therapy" or counseling. Hopefully the patient will accommodate to his disability and better integrate his desires and his abilities. However, irritability is a common manifestation of depression, so that must be factored in when making any assessment.

A 56-year-old man is referred to a psychiatrist after his primary care physician (PCP) treats him with two different antidepressants that are unhelpful. The patient denies feeling depressed, although he readily admits to feeling sluggish and fatigued. A complete evaluation by the PCP found nothing abnormal to explain the fatigue and slowness. In addition the patient "looks" depressed and his voice is softer and less expressive. He can't get comfortable in bed so his sleeping has become poor, and work has become more of a chore than an enjoyment, which it once was.

The tremor of PD is present in 80% of PD patients, so that 20% don't have it. When the tremor is absent, the diagnosis of PD is frequently not made and patients may be mistakenly diagnosed as being depressed based on the physical changes due to PD.

Depression is common in PD. In fact, it is generally considered to be the single most common psychiatric problem in the disease. In most studies, depending on a variety of factors I'll discuss below, depression affects between 10% and 90% of PD patients, although a figure of 40% to 50% is probably more accurate. However, what we mean when we use the term "depression" is itself unclear in PD. Depression in the "normal" population is subdivided into a variety of subtypes, just as cancer, or even types of cancer, such as skin cancer, is subdivided into a host of categories. Each is defined differently, perhaps treated differently, and each may have a different course. Although lay people think of depression as being synonymous with sadness, this is not always the case. Psychiatrists will often refer to "melancholic depression," meaning depression with sadness, or to "nonmelancholic depression," which is a depression without profound sadness.

O*ver the past few months, Ms. S. has become very withdrawn. She cries sometimes for no apparent reason. And even though she's in better shape than most of her elderly friends, despite her PD, she feels that life isn't worth living. She feels sad most of the day, every day. She's given up socializing. She eats only if forced to. She sleeps poorly but spends more than 12 hours in bed.*

This is a patient with a major depression.

"Major depression" involves the presence of at least five of nine symptoms. All need to have been present for two weeks or longer and not to have been present for months. They must cause significant distress or a decline in function. One of the five symptoms must include either sadness or loss of enjoyment or interest in things that formerly were pleasurable. The three or four other symptoms must include weight change (loss or gain), sleep disorders, agitation or retardation, fatigue (loss of energy), feelings of worthlessness or guilt, reduced concentration and decision making, and suicidal thoughts. The other forms of depression generally involve having fewer symptoms, and the symptoms are less severe.

The difficulty in diagnosing depression in PD is that many of the symptoms of depression are the same as the motor problems of PD that even the most nondepressed PD patients have. In fact, one of my patients told me that the PD symptom that bothered him the most, during the first few years of his PD, was not his rather prominent tremor but his facial expression. He told me that he felt fine, but all his acquaintances would ask his wife, "Why is Don so depressed?" He was annoyed that his "masked facial expression" belied his actual mood.

Aside from the core question—what is the person's actual mood?—we run into confounding issues. PD patients often lose weight due to their PD, whether they're depressed or not. Some PD patients have swallowing problems so they only eat soft, easy-to-swallow foods that may not be appetizing. Other PD patients eat so slowly that they are self-conscious about taking so long and have reduced the amount they eat for social purposes. Meanwhile, some PD patients gain a lot of weight either because they've stopped exercising or because they take medications that increase their appetite.

Many PD patients lose interest in hobbies or recreations that formerly brought great pleasure but now are mainly seen as frustrating. The difficulty of sailing a boat, playing golf, drawing pictures, fixing the house, knitting, cooking, singing or playing music, doing crossword puzzles, and heaven knows what else now causes more grief than pleasure. Even the difficulty of engaging in conversation when it's difficult for people to hear what the PD patient is saying dramatically reduces the enjoyment that social gatherings once brought. While "slowing down" (psychomotor retardation) is a cardinal feature of depression in the general population, it is obviously one of the central problems in PD. To think that someone who is slow is therefore depressed, is similar to thinking that someone with a masked facial expression must be depressed because he looks depressed.

Many PD patients are first diagnosed with depression before the PD is appreciated. This is actually one of the problems doctors have had over the years, trying to sort out the "chicken-and-egg" problem I began the chapter with. Do the symptoms of PD cause the depression or is the depression one of the symptoms of PD, like tremor and slowness? One of the arguments in favor of depression being intrinsic to the disease, that it is a direct result of the loss of brain cells, has been that the depression sometimes precedes the diagnosis. The argument goes as follows: if the depression occurs before the person knows he has PD, then the depression can't be reactive. The problem with that answer is twofold. First of all, many people are diagnosed with depression *because* the symptoms of PD are mistaken for depression, even when they're not depressed. The family and the doctors see the reduced facial expression, the slowness, the quiet voice and assume the person is depressed, and only when the tremor appears do the gears shift and suddenly the person has PD, is treated with medicines for PD, and a lot of the "depression" vanishes.

In other words many people, especially if they lack the typical rest tremor, are diagnosed with depression when they really have PD. These patients actually have "pseudodepression," that is, a false depression. They look depressed but aren't. The second answer to the observation that many people are diagnosed with depression before PD is that as PD sets in, certain things become harder to do and everything takes longer. Fatigue may set in, and over the course of a year or so the person starts feeling old. Life becomes a series of frustrations as "the old get-up-and-go got up and went." So, in this context, when PD has not been diagnosed and all the medical work-ups have been unrevealing, the person, feeling frustrated, having symptoms that overlap greatly with PD, is diagnosed with depression when the real diagnosis is "frustration."

Sleep disorders are common in depression, both problems falling asleep and problems staying asleep. However, as most people with PD know, they too have problems with sleep whether they are depressed or not (see Chapter 12). In a nutshell, people with PD have difficulty getting comfortable in order to fall asleep. They frequently have pain. They can't turn over. The tremor keeps them awake. They can't get their head to lie comfortably on the pillow. They're anxious and stay awake worrying about all sorts of things, whether they're worth worrying about or not. Then once they're asleep they awaken because their bladder is hyperactive. The tremor wakes them up. They napped for two hours during the day so they don't need much sleep at night. They yell or laugh in their sleep, which also wakes them up. They act out a dream and punch the headboard, causing them to awaken. And on and on. In depression there is a classic observation, called early morning awakening. Depressed people frequently sleep through the night but awaken an hour or more before they want or need to and can't fall back to sleep. In PD it is unknown if this occurs because PD patients wake up so often during the night, and sometimes awaken purposefully an hour or two before they intend to actually get up so that they can take their PD medications in order to "turn on" before they get out of bed.

Fatigue, or loss of energy, is very common in PD, whether the patients are depressed or not. Fatigue is common in virtually all medical disorders—anemia, infections of all types, heart failure, obstructive lung disease, kidney failure, lupus, cancer, you name it. So it too cannot necessarily be used to diagnose PD.

The difficulty in diagnosing depression in PD was actually the subject of a small National Institutes of Health conference in 2004, bringing together experts on geriatric psychiatry and specialists in PD, trying to hone in simply on how to make the diagnosis. This is important for several reasons, including how to know if a treatment is working. To define a treatment as a success there has to be a way to measure the outcome.

When I think about how I make the diagnosis of depression in someone with PD I think of Supreme Court Justice Stewart's famous statement concerning pornography, "I know it when I see it." For the nonpsychiatrist it is important to realize that not everyone who meets the criteria for a diagnosis of depression feels sad. If you look at the following table, with the criteria for a diagnosis of major depression, it is clear that the patient must have one of two cardinal features, and only one of them is sadness. Loss of pleasure or interest is the other. Unfortunately, many people with PD develop apathy (see Chapter 4). Therefore apathetic PD patients are often mistaken for depressed

• • • • • • • • • • MAJOR DEPRESSIVE DISORDER • • • • • • • • •

A. Five or more of the following occurring during a two-week
    period and a change from previous functioning. Either
    #1 or #2 must be present:
    1. depressed mood most of the day, nearly every day
    2. markedly diminished interest or pleasure most of the
        day, nearly every day

B. Four of the following must also be present:
    3. significant weight gain or loss without a diet
    4. insomnia or hypersomnia nearly every day
    5. psychomotor agitation or retardation nearly every day
    6. fatigue nearly every day
    7. feelings of worthlessness or excessive or inappropriate
        guilt nearly every day
    8. diminished ability to think or concentrate, or
        indecisiveness nearly every day
    9. recurrent thoughts of death, or recurrent suicidal
        ideation

C. The symptoms cause distress or impairment
D. The symptoms aren't directly due to drugs or a
    physiological disorder
E. The symptoms are not due to bereavement

• •

Based on *The Diagnostic and Statistical Manual of Mental Disorders, IV-TR,* created
by the American Psychiatric Association to define all psychiatric disorders.

PD patients. After all, they've lost interest and pleasure in almost
everything around them.

I don't think there is any ideal way to decide if a PD patient is
depressed. I believe that even experts may see the same patient and
come to different conclusions about whether the patient is depressed
or not. I consider the patient's mood as the single most important indicator. Does the patient feel sad, blue, depressed? If yes, is it a sustained
feeling? After all, every normal person feels sad once in a while, or
even more than that. Does this feeling of sadness interfere with the
person's usual lifestyle?

Diminished interest is another symptom that could be due to depression or to the motor dysfunction of PD. If golf or tennis was a hobby that was at the center of a person's life, then it may not be so easy to give up. Many hobbies such as these not only provide pleasure in and of themselves but also provide social rewards. Getting together once or twice a week with the "boys" or "girls" for an afternoon of golf, then becoming unable to play the game, also brings about a change in socialization. Sometimes life centers on a job that can't be done, making alterations in the house, singing in church, or any number of vocations that can no longer be done at all, or are performed in such a way that the activity itself becomes heartbreaking to even approach. Even something as nonphysically demanding as reading can become difficult, whether from tremor, difficulty turning a page, difficulty staying awake, or soft speech, making discussion of the book with others problematic.

Fatigue is so common that there is a whole chapter of this book devoted to it. Although it is more common among depressed people with PD according to some studies (but not all), it is also seen in people who are not depressed. On rare occasion people have gone to the doctor because of unexplained fatigue and then were diagnosed with PD. Interestingly, the fatigue is not related to the degree of motor impairment and thus appears to be a symptom of the PD itself, present both in the young PD patient with only minimum disability, as well as the older, advanced PD patient who spends the day in the wheelchair expending very little energy.

Many people with PD feel guilty about how much their illness has affected their loved ones. Instead of traveling the world, spending afternoons playing bridge or golf, taking cruises twice a year, babysitting the grandchildren, they have dragged down their spouse into a caregiver's role. Sometimes a child becomes the caregiver, having to give up the extra income of a job, his or her own retirement time, and so on. While it's obvious that no one is to "blame" for this, it doesn't alter the basic fact that this illness happened to one person and this person has now altered others' lives.

Altered concentration can be so intrinsic to any sleep disturbance, which itself is so common in PD that it is difficult to include this symptom in defining depression. Of course, as with the others, it's applied in a practical fashion. Is the impaired concentration due to the mood change or is it due to sleepiness or possibly to medications? In addition, some patients are thought by others to be indecisive simply because their speech has become soft or slurred so that its previous decisiveness may have been lost. In other cases, a very independent person now has to make decisions that involve others and no longer feels decisive because she is so reliant on others. Another problem that may cloud the interpretation of this symptom is that some PD patients develop memory or cognitive impairments that inhibit their decision-making capabilities. Suicide is very uncommon in PD.

Item C in the table on depression (see page 54) requires either distress or impairment. If distress is present and the distress is thought to be due to the mood rather than the frustration of the PD motor disability, then the diagnosis of depression is easy. However the patient and the family frequently cannot distinguish the cause of the distress since all the problems are so closely intertwined. The same is true for disabilities. Is the patient impaired because of his slow, hypophonic (soft) speech, is it the frustration he feels in not being able to communicate, or is it the sense of futility he feels, that life has closed in and limited him (i.e., depression)?

WHICH COMES FIRST, THE CHICKEN OR THE EGG?

Recent observations have proven that depression sometimes occurs as "part" of PD and not simply as a "reaction" to the disease. One of the early recipients of a deep brain stimulator for treating the motor problems in PD developed an overwhelming depression within seconds of having the stimulator turned on. When the choice of which electrodes to stimulate was altered, the stimulation did not cause this problem, and the patient had never had significant problems with depression before. Each time the stimulator was turned on using certain electrodes, the patient instantly became severely depressed, and each time the stimulator was turned off the depression lifted. This demonstrated quite clearly that there are pathways deep in the brain, some of them associated with PD, that clearly influence mood. And although deep brain stimulation obviously doesn't occur naturally in PD, very closely related circuits are definitely involved in PD. This issue has been important in our understanding of the brain.

A famous study performed in the 1970s compared depression in patients with PD to patients with rheumatoid arthritis (RA). RA was chosen because it has many similarities to PD. Both are progressive, disabling, and incurable although there are medications that can improve the symptoms. They both affect walking and dexterity, and PD was thought at that time to not significantly affect memory or thinking. The interesting outcome of that study was the observation that both groups were about equally affected by depression. This study then suggested that depression was likely to be a reaction to the disability of PD and less likely to be "intrinsic," that is, part of the disease itself, like tremor. Other observations about depression in PD suggested that there were differences between depression in PD and non-PD groups, that PD patients were less likely to feel guilty, for example, but the data for these studies were quite small, and although possibly true, not convincing yet.

WHEN IS A PD PATIENT DEPRESSED?

So, what does it mean for a PD patient to be depressed? I think it is unclear. This means that different doctors may well disagree about whether a patient is depressed or not. I think of depression as primarily reflecting a mood of sadness that is beyond what the person's personality and circumstances would lead me to expect. This mood change causes pain either for the patient or for those around him, and adds to the general level of dysfunction and distress caused by the PD and its motor consequences. An important point is that even in depressed patients the mood is not always sad. Sometimes the depression manifests itself as withdrawal or irritability. I think that when in doubt, assume that the problem is, in fact, part of a depression and then treat it to see if it responds.

A 50-year-old woman has had PD for four years. Her husband left the family one year before her diagnosis. Her teenage son is in trouble with the police and her daughter has a child but no relationship with the father of the child. The patient can't sleep at night, worried about her troubled family and paying the next mortgage installment. She feels overwhelmed, but denies suicidality, or feelings of sadness. She thinks, "things will work out."

This patient, despite overwhelming problems, is not depressed.

A 68-year-old man has withdrawn from his family. He sits by the window all day watching traffic. His conversations are limited to single words, if at all possible. He easily loses his temper, and rarely smiles, but denies feeling depressed.

This patient probably is depressed. While he might be apathetic, the fact that he is irritable suggests that he is not without mood. He apparently does care about something, suggesting that his withdrawal is not passive, but an active method of dealing with his emotional crisis.

TREATMENT

All PD specialists believe that treatment for depression in PD is not different than for other populations with depression. Since the first edition of this book two significant studies have finally shown that depression does in fact respond to antidepressant medications. One study evaluated pramipexole, a dopamine agonist, which is used to treat the motor symptoms of PD and found that it elevated mood in depressed PD patients. Through some statistical manipulations, the authors were able to demonstrate that the depression was independent of the improvement in motor function. Unfortunately, while the improvement was statistically significant, it was not large enough to be very significant from a clinical vantage point. A second study compared two "standard" antidepressants, paroxetine (Paxil) and venlafaxine (Effexor), to placebo and found that both were helpful, both clinically and statistically. Presumably these results extend to other similar drugs, even though they were not tested. While this is good news, there was some bad news associated with this study as well. The first bit of bad news was that although the results were "significant," they were not robust. Many patients did not improve. The second bit of bad news was that the study was stopped only halfway through because the investigators couldn't recruit enough subjects. So, even though depression affects almost half of the PD population, most centers in the study, all of which had huge PD populations, couldn't recruit more than one or two subjects per year! It is not known if this poor showing was due to many patients already being on treatment, and therefore not eligible to join the study, or to patients being unwilling to participate. Most likely the answer is a mixture of both explanations.

There is no consensus among doctors on how best to treat depression. Quite clearly some people will respond better to one medication or another, just as some will develop side effects of one and not another. Nonpharmacologic approaches have not been adequately studied, so the effect of the "talking cure" is unknown in PD although it is known to be as helpful as medication in non-PD patients. Thus, we do not know if some sort of psychotherapy is helpful or not in PD. It is hard to imagine that exercise, good sleep habits, and regular social interactions aren't good for improving mood, just as they are in the general population. A form of psychotherapy called cognitive behavior therapy (CBT) shows promise but is time intensive.

Most PD specialists use antidepressants, but it is unclear if certain ones are better than others. The only large, multicentered study showed that paroxetine and venlafaxine were helpful, and most doctors think this means that it is likely that all antidepressants are helpful, but this is not known, and most of these medications will never be studied.

Some antidepressants have side effects that sometimes can be put to advantage in PD. For example, the chemical class of the older antidepressants, the tricyclics, often cause dry mouth and reduced bladder function, which can be helpful in PD. Mirtazepine (Remeron) is very sedating, increases appetite, and sometimes helps tremor in PD. For certain people, particularly thin ones with tremor who sleep poorly at night, this can be a great drug. Bupropion, which is used both to treat depression and to reduce the urge to smoke cigarettes, may be useful in some PD patients as well. In short, there are reasons to favor one drug over another, but these reasons are all relative, and none are supported by data. It is probably wisest, therefore, for the treating doctor to choose whichever drug he feels most comfortable with.

ELECTROCONVULSIVE THERAPY

Although electroconvulsive therapy (ECT), shock therapy, has gotten a bad rap, it is the single most effective treatment for depression in the general population. ECT consists of a series of brain seizures induced by an electrical shock applied to the scalp. The patient is anesthetized and paralyzed just as in minor surgery so that nothing is remembered. The shock produces an electrical seizure in the brain but does not produce a convulsion of the body because of the paralyzing drug. Therefore the patient awakens later without the aches and pains that epileptic seizures produce. Typically patients receive a series of eight to twelve seizures, usually given two or three per week, spaced out so that there are rest days in between. Sustained improvement in mood generally begins to occur by the eighth seizure.

There is a good news/bad news side to ECT in PD. The good news is that many patients, perhaps most, enjoy improvement in motor function, sometimes dramatic improvement, starting even before the improvement in the depression. The bad news is that all patients experience a delirious state after the seizure, and this confusional state may last several hours to even a few days in an elderly PD patient with some memory problems. While most patients do not recall this delirium, there are occasional patients who report a permanent mild memory deficit from their ECT. This memory problem has never been documented with formal neuropsychological testing. All testing has shown that memory returns to normal, but nevertheless some patients do report chronic low-level memory impairments.

Once the patient improves with ECT, antidepressant medication is begun. Typically, these patients did not respond to antidepressants before the ECT, or else they would not have been given the ECT. After ECT, however, when the depression has improved or remitted, the antidepressants work. Some patients, with particularly difficult-to-treat depression may require "maintenance ECT." This refers to regular single seizures induced every three to six weeks, usually about once each month.

Most neurologists shy away from ECT, even PD specialists, because neurologists are all trained to think of seizures as bad for the brain. In addition, American culture is schooled in the belief that ECT is barbaric and used partially as punishment, as shown in the movie, *One Flew over the Cuckoo's Nest*, where Jack Nicholson is given ECT to punish him for undermining the evil nurse's grip on the ward. Berkeley, California, actually banned ECT in that city.

Some psychiatrists who specialize in ECT have suggested that ECT is so effective in improving the motor aspects of PD even as it improves depression that ECT should be tested as a treatment for the motor aspects of PD. This idea has no traction among neurologists or others who specialize in PD.

Here is a true anecdote: an 80-year-old man who had suffered with PD for over 15 years was crying in my office. His PD was quite severe. He needed help to stand up from a chair. He drooled constantly, which embarrassed him greatly. Walking was poor but he could ambulate without assistance. I thought that his memory was impaired, but it was difficult to tell because his emotional distress was so severe. "I want to die. I can't go on like this." He failed trials of different antidepressants, so I arranged to have a psychiatrist evaluate him for

ECT. He was admitted to the psychiatric hospital and I visited him. When I walked on the ward I saw him sitting in a chair, wearing a brightly colored Hawaiian shirt, reading a magazine. He saw me, smiled broadly and stood up. "Dr. Friedman, it's nice to see you." "You look terrific," I said. I was stunned. Not just that he looked so wonderful but also that he not only recognized me, but recalled my name. He put his arm around my shoulder and told me, "This place is great. Every morning a nurse takes off my clothes, washes me all over, puts powder all over and then dresses me. Then they bring me food. This place is great." I was impressed by how dramatic this response to ECT had been. I inquired about how many treatments the patient had received. The amazing answer was, "None." He had not been treated in any way! It appears that just admitting him to the hospital, giving him the special care he evidently needed, was enough to reclaim his poor soul. After a few days without other treatments, his mood remained remarkably positive, and he was discharged without getting ECT or other treatments. I saw him in the office a few weeks later. He needed help to get up from the chair. He was drooling horribly. His speech was difficult to understand. "I want to die. I can't go on like this."

Here was an example of someone whose mood depended on a variety of external needs that couldn't be provided. Although he seemed quite clearly depressed to me, his sadness was due to the misfit between his needs and his ability to adjust to getting old, having an elderly and infirm wife, and his severe parkinsonism. The interaction between his mood and his motor function was amazing. When he felt good he moved as he had five years earlier. When he felt good he thought as he had ten years earlier. He was a new man, but only on the psychiatry ward, not in "real life" at home. He remained a broken man who we couldn't "fix." He exemplifies the extremely complex nature of the interactions between the "mind" and the motor functions of the brain, which are so common in this disease.

6

Anxiety

Excess anxiety may affect up to 40% of people with Parkinson's disease (PD). It is frequently associated with depression (making both conditions worse), psychosis, or other behavioral problems, but it also may exist on its own. "Anxiety disorders" refer to a set of complex problems. Although anxiety means nervousness, "anxiety disorders" encompass several syndromes related to the core problem of nervousness. Since anxiety is common in people without PD or any other medical condition and also complicates several mental disorders, this chapter will begin with a review of anxiety disorders in general before focusing on PD.

Since publication of the first edition of this book, I have come to a heightened appreciation for the importance of anxiety disorders in PD. Certainly I knew it was a significant problem, but in recent years I've encountered an increasing number of people whose anxiety is so severe that it dwarfs the motor problems of PD and tortures the patients even more than hallucinations and delusions. And, in a manner unlike the other behavior problems of PD, anxiety causes afflicted patients to bother everyone around them.

WHAT ARE ANXIETY DISORDERS?

Anxiety is a natural human condition. It is impossible to lead any sort of lifestyle without some occasional degree of nervousness. Anxiety is generally an uncomfortable feeling that something bad is going to happen. It is frequently accompanied by physiological changes such as rapid heartbeat, rapid breathing, sweating, or diarrhea. In many cases this is a healthy response to a situation. For example, driving at night in a blizzard with poor visibility should induce anxiety; being in a combat zone; investing a mortgage payment in a "surefire" stock; singing one's first solo with a church choir; taking an important test. The list is endless. All of these make most people anxious and we would wonder about the person who wasn't nervous in these situations. While we might think a person has "nerves of steel," we might also think the person was not reacting properly. "Foolhardy" is a term used to describe someone who is not appropriately anxious.

M*r. S. had been a fairly serious man, not given to excessive worry, until he turned 68, three years after he retired. He began to worry about his retirement account although, as his wife pointed out, their finances were in very good health and hadn't changed. He also worried after every snowstorm whether the mailman would be able to make deliveries, although there were no special items expected. A year later he developed a resting tremor.*

Anxiety *disorders* refer to nervous conditions that are inappropriate to the situation and therefore are maladaptive. The anxiety is either magnified beyond what is considered appropriate, or the anxiety is irrational. A person who faints or becomes mute when asked to talk in public would have an exaggerated degree of anxiety. Being anxious is normal in that situation, but not to the extent of being incapacitated. Panicking and screaming because one is in a small space, due to claustrophobia, is an example of an irrational response, a form of anxiety based on no explainable threat.

A 60-year-old man sees the doctor because of slowness using his right arm. He is sent for an MRI, but once he's in the tube he panics and starts screaming to let him out.

Anxiety disorders are common in the general population, but are much increased in PD. They appear to be part of the illness itself, not just a reaction to the uncertainties of the disease. Men and women are equally affected by anxiety, whereas in the general population, anxiety is far more common in women. And the age of the onset for anxiety is considerably older when it occurs in PD than when it occurs in the general population.

Anxiety in PD is poorly understood. People generally become "nervous" for no apparent reason. It is due to a biochemical abnormality in the brain. It is part of the PD, just like tremor, rigidity, and slowness. Since anxiety tends to be relatively constant we tend to think of anxiety as being more like a personality trait, rather than as an illness or chemical brain imbalance. We think of certain people as being "nervous types," or "nervous Nellies," rather than thinking of them as having a *behavioral disorder*. And, of course, where "normal" ends and "abnormal" begins is often not at all clear.

DISORDERS THAT LOOK LIKE ANXIETY

There are other types of "nervous disorders" that have the same or similar symptoms and can be mistaken for generalized anxiety. Restlessness and L-Dopa–induced dyskinesias can look like anxiety. Restlessness, called "akathisia," is a common problem in PD. It is also a common problem with restless legs syndrome, which may occur in

• • • • • • • • DISORDERS THAT MAY LOOK LIKE • • • • • • •
ANXIETY IN PD PATIENTS

Akathisia—the syndrome of motor restlessness
Restless legs syndrome
L-Dopa–induced dyskinesias
Withdrawal from alcohol or narcotics (unrelated to PD)
Pain-induced restlessness and distractibility
Rapid breathing with or without shortness of breath due to
        L-Dopa or PD itself
Fever
Medication or drug effect

• •

PD. Restlessnes is also a side effect of some drugs or drug withdrawal, particularly alcohol.

TYPES OF ANXIETY DISORDERS

In the general population there are nine subtypes of anxiety disorders, but only a few are of interest to us. Most lay people, and non-psychiatric physicians too, think of *generalized anxiety disorder* (GAD, overanxious) as what we mean when we think about anxiety as a problem, but some PD patients develop phobias (irrational fears) or panic disorder. Obsessive–compulsive disorder is classified as an anxiety disorder but will be discussed in a separate chapter.

Anxiety frequently accompanies "wearing off," when PD drugs start to lose their efficacy, but also may fluctuate through the day, without any apparent relationship to motor function or drug schedule. Anxiety is also commonly present with depression. People who are dependent on some drugs may start feeling anxious when they are "due" for their next dose (a type of wearing off). This may be especially true for drugs of addiction such as alcohol, stimulants, and narcotics, whether taken for pain or to get "high." Some people who drink too many caffeinated beverages also get restless or jittery and may appear anxious.

• • • • • • • GENERALIZED ANXIETY DISORDER • • • • • • •
(OVERANXIOUS SYNDROME)

1. Excessive anxiety and worry about several things on most
    days occurring for at least six months
2. The nervousness is hard to control and is associated with at
    least three of the following problems:
    Restlessness or feeling "on edge"
    Fatigue
    Poor concentration
    Irritability
    Muscle tension
    Sleep problems

• •

GENERALIZED ANXIETY DISORDER

The most common type of anxiety problem that PD patients have is GAD, also called "overanxious disorder." The above table describes the problem.

Given that anxiety is common in PD and that PD is common in general, it is quite surprising that there have been few studies of this problem in PD. In many cases the anxiety is a lifelong problem that has nothing to do with the PD, but in many cases anxiety develops late in life just preceding the development or the recognition of the PD itself.

In one study in the United States, patients with PD and controls (people who did not have PD) of the same age were compared on an anxiety scale. The PD patients, on average, had a significantly higher score. It is impossible to say how much of the anxiety is "reactive," just due to having the problems that come with PD, and how much is a direct result of the brain changes. In relatively small studies anxiety appears to affect between 5% and 40% of the people surveyed. This is in striking contrast to the prevalence of anxiety in the general American population. In a survey of close to 20,000 Americans over the age of 65, only about 5% were found to have anxiety.

Anxiety may be medication related. All the medications that are useful in PD work either directly or indirectly on the brain, and the dopamine system is involved in many behaviors and emotions. One study reported that almost one-quarter of the patients developed anxiety when a dopamine agonist was added to their medication regimen. Another study directly contradicted this and found no increase in anxiety in patients who took the exact same drug. These sorts of conflicting studies are the reason more, and larger, studies are needed.

In some patients the anxiety develops only during "off" periods, that is, when the PD medications stop working and the patient loses mobility. Many patients, despite suffering through these episodes thousands of times, still feel as if they're never going to snap out of it and become extremely anxious whenever their medications stop working. And, of course, as it is well known that nervousness causes PD symptoms to worsen, a vicious cycle develops. Because this is a disorder, and not under voluntary control, the anxiety is irrational and not curable simply by reassurance.

Although most PD patients who suffer from anxiety develop the overanxious type, all of the anxiety disorders have been reported in PD.

Anxiety in PD does not correlate with severity of the motor disability. It is therefore not true, in general, that anxiety worsens as the disease progresses or that the more severely affected patients are likely to be the most anxious. Although it has not been adequately studied, I believe that anxiety is more common in patients who suffer clinical fluctuations, and not just when the patient is in the "off" state. Thus, I believe that anxiety occurs either as a feature of the PD itself, sometimes predating the onset of symptoms or of diagnosis, but also develops during the course of the disease, and then it typically occurs in people who fluctuate, or in people who have sudden worsening of their motor function, especially in public situations, which is one of the features of social phobias, another anxiety disorder.

In my experience patients are so bedeviled by the problems that develop when their medications stop working adequately, that they worry all the time about these "off" periods. In other words, I think there are more PD patients who are anxious that they will turn "off" than there are those who become anxious only when they are in or entering an "off" condition. The unpredictability of their ability to perform their day's chores or social events is simply devastating and anxiety provoking.

Although many PD specialists have been impressed that anxiety seems to go hand-in-hand with clinical fluctuators, people being anxious when "off" and feeling fine when "on," further studies have found that most PD patients with anxiety do not, in fact, fluctuate with their motor capabilities. This means that many PD patients will have "on" and "off" periods and, in addition, have anxious and nonanxious periods, and the two may not have anything to do with each other. This implies that getting the motor fluctuations under control may not have a great impact on the anxiety.

ANXIETY AND DEPRESSION

In one comparison between PD patients and their spouses, 20% of PD patients who had either depression or anxiety had both at the same time. This was a rare coincidence in the spouse group. In addition the presence of the two problems together is about twice that recorded in the general population in other studies. Another study reported that over 90% of anxiety-stricken PD patients also had depression or symptoms of depression.

A 65-year-old man becomes increasingly sad, tired and inattentive. He worries that something bad is going to happen to his wife so he refuses to let her out of his sight. When she goes to another room, he keeps questioning whoever is with him, "Do you think something's happened to her? Do you think she's OK? Let's go check on her."

ANXIETY COMPLICATING OTHER BEHAVIORAL PROBLEMS

Anxiety occurs with dementia and psychosis. The problem that doctors have in treating this is that it is difficult to figure out which problem is the "main" one and which makes the other worse. As doctors, we often tend to think that one problem is "driving" the other, by which we mean that the anxiety, for example, makes the depression or psychosis worse by pushing or magnifying it. In such cases it is sometimes worthwhile to treat the anxiety in order to lessen the severity of the other condition.

A 79-year-old woman begins to see children in her house who aren't real. She becomes preoccupied with the well-being of these children, repeatedly asking where their mothers are and why no one has come to pick them up. She worries that the police may come and arrest her for kidnapping.

In this case the psychotic symptoms, hallucinations, are fueling the anxiety by providing a concrete situation to focus on.

PHYSIOLOGICAL ASPECTS OF ANXIETY

Anxiety is associated with significant physiological dysfunction. Parkinson symptoms all worsen with anxiety. Speech worsens for those with a speech problem. Tremors always worsen with nervousness, and, interestingly, dyskinesias also get worse with anxiety. This is interesting because tremors indicate a medication under-effect while dyskinesias indicate a medication over-effect. So, whether under- or over-medicated, anxiety causes whichever movements are in excess to worsen. Generally, whatever problems you have at the moment are amplified by anxiety.

• • • • • • • • • • • • • PANIC DISORDER • • • • • • • • • • • • •

Recurrent unexpected spells, without apparent precipitant, in
which at least four of the following occur:
Palpitations
Sweating
Trembling or shaking
Shortness of breath
Feeling of choking/shortness of breath
Chest pain or discomfort
Nausea or abdominal distress
Dizziness, feeling lightheaded or faint
Derealization (the sensation that things are not real)
or depersonalization
Fear of becoming "out of control" or "crazy"
Fear of dying
Numbness or tingling
Chills or hot flashes

• •

A 73-year-old man avoids restaurants because he freezes whenever he enters one. He worries about socializing with his friends and often avoids them because they frequently end their socializing by going to a restaurant.

INNER TREMOR

Many patients suffer from a sensation that they are shaking internally. In a high percentage of cases this tremor is experienced in a part of the body that can't actually tremor. Patients may experience their chest or abdomen shaking despite being fully aware that no tremor can be seen. Sometimes they will feel that their limbs are shaking even though they can see that they are not. Nevertheless, patients are convinced that the shaking is real. Until I read about this peculiar, yet common problem, I assumed that this was a "forme fruste" of a tremor, in other words, the patient was very sensitive and could feel that a tremor was developing before it could be seen. However this was usually not the case, and when I recognized that this was something different and started asking my patients about it, I learned that they knew if they had an "inner" tremor or a visible tremor. I used to sometimes treat this sensation of tremor as if it was a real tremor, using the same drugs that we use to treat tremor in PD, and they never worked. It turns out that the sensation of an inner tremor is most closely linked to anxiety. It is, to a large extent, a symptom of "nerves." The treatment of this is therefore with medications for anxiety, and not medications for the PD.

A 58-year-old man complains of bothersome tremor but is not shaking in the office. "I don't have it now," he reports, "but at home it's real bad." It turns out that the tremor is in his chest and that no one can see it.

MANAGEMENT

There are virtually no studies on the treatment of anxiety in PD. While there is no reason to think that PD patients will respond any differently from other people of the same age, there are reasons to think that side effects will be considerably more common. The anti-anxiety drugs fall into two broad categories.

The newer generation of antidepressants, the selective serotonin reuptake inhibitor (SSRI) drugs, not only treat depression but also treat anxiety. They work more quickly for anxiety than depression, but they can't be taken on an as-needed basis, that is, they can't be taken when the patient feels anxious because they take weeks to work.

In the other class are mostly chemical relatives of diazepam (Valium). The same drugs are used to treat insomnia. Obviously they cause sedation. In addition, studies of these drugs in the elderly indicate a clear increase in the risk of falling, For someone with PD who already has balance problems, adding a drug that may worsen balance is an obvious problem. These drugs also may cause some degree of confusion. So, the antianxiety drugs may increase daytime sleepiness, increase the risk of falling, and increase the risk of developing halluci- nations and confusion.

On the other hand, the drugs are extremely safe medically. They work in minutes to hours. They do not suppress breathing, so that there is almost no chance of a fatal or serious overdose. And it is often not appreciated that if a patient sleeps through the night her balance and gait may actually improve, not worsen, and hallucinations and confusion may also improve so that these drugs may *improve* the PD. Because anxiety worsens PD symptoms, treating the anxiety may indirectly improve motor function, not worsen it. I believe, therefore, that there is no absolute rule on treatment.

When psychosis and anxiety occur together, the management is more difficult because the antipsychotic drugs are, like the antianxi- ety drugs, sedating. The combination of the two types of drugs may simply put the patient to sleep and make him delirious when awake, basically in a drug fog. On the other hand, some of the antipsychotics also treat anxiety.

One of the most bothersome set of problems for PD patients is the development of anxiety associated with bodily symptoms. In some cases the bodily symptoms are clearly psychotic in nature. A man wants to go to the hospital because he knows he is about to die because his lungs aren't working. Yet he's not short of breath. Another day he believes that he cannot eat because his stomach stopped working. More common however is the patient who reports gastrointestinal problems, rectal pain, abdominal pressure, and peculiar sensations in the abdo- men that fit no physiological explanation and for which no diagnostic test finds any suggestion of a cause. This is not a rare problem for the severely anxious, and, as you would expect, the anxiety makes the abdominal symptoms worse, which then make the anxiety worse.

Meanwhile, the gastroenterologist has explained that there are no more tests that can be done and that there is no medical explana- tion. And there isn't, in the sense of "internal medicine." But this is not a very rare problem among the anxious. Its recognition is extremely important because the poor patient is suffering and making those around him suffer as well. Between trips to the doctor, the emergency room, the radiology suite, the enemas, the belittling comments from the emergency room staff, the problem becomes catastrophic.

My psychiatric colleagues and I have recently had some success using electroconvulsive therapy (ECT) for this, a treatment not widely accepted for treating severe anxiety, but something that I believe should be considered in extreme cases.

7

· ·

Dementia

Dementia means a permanent decline in memory and thinking skills sufficient to cause a problem in everyday functioning. It is the worst of the problems that may occur in Parkinson's disease (PD). Luckily, when it does develop, it does not affect most PD patients until late in the course. Unfortunately, it is a common problem. It is different from Alzheimer's disease (AD), but shares several of its characteristics, particularly the memory failure.

Dementia is a multifaceted problem because it causes more than the memory problem. People with dementia are more likely to die sooner, develop hallucinations and delusions on the usual PD medications, become depressed, become apathetic, become anxious, and develop sleep disorders. This is undoubtedly due to the fact that dementia occurs only when large numbers of brain cells, distributed over a large region begin to deteriorate and die. Many of these regions are involved in more than one thought or emotional process and when the cells deteriorate, several brain processes are affected.

Memory impairment is a somewhat hazy concept. Older adults frequently experience "senior moments" when they forget things, particularly names, that are so deeply entrenched in their memory banks that they never thought they would forget them.

We sometimes find a bend in the road unfamiliar even though we've driven the route daily for decades. We forget important conversations, birthdates, and so on. Neurologists frequently evaluate middle-aged and older people, self-referred because of the fear that they have AD. In general, people who think they have Alzheimer's don't, while those who do have it often lack the insight to recognize they have a problem, and deny their increasing difficulties. It is normal to forget. In addition, although we (hopefully) get wiser with age, we do not get smarter. And our memories don't get better either. In fact, the scores on IQ tests are graded in such a way that the elderly get higher scores with more errors and fewer correct answers, that is, older people have worse memories and problem-solving skills than younger adults. Therefore, although an IQ of 100 means "normal," the score of 100 means something different for a 25-year-old and a 75-year-old. This is an important concept, because much of the neurology of older people involves "clinical judgment" to distinguish abnormal from normal in some older people. Memory and thinking skills deteriorate with age just as athletic skills do.

Not all memory problems are permanent. Depression, anxiety, and sleep disorders also cause memory to worsen. If one thinks that physical pain causes people to concentrate, think, and remember less well, then one can think of depression and anxiety as causing psychic pain that also interferes with memory and cognition. Memory problems fall into two main categories: absence of a memory trace and problems with memory access. If one imagines a "memory bank" as being like a blackboard or a page where something is written down, then there is a memory failure if the blackboard or page is blank because the memory was never written down or it is erased. It is a different problem if the memory is written but the proper page cannot be located. If someone is in pain he will not pay attention, and therefore not register a memory. Thus, there is no memory trace, no stored memory. The blackboard is clean. If a person fails to pay attention, then memories do not get stored. There are huge numbers of reasons for this, from depression and anxiety, to pain, sleepiness and boredom. Just think of all those teachers who tried to teach you things that just sailed in one ear and out the other. So, memory failures are commonly due to poor attention. How many spouses have gone to the market to buy a small number of items, only to forget the one or two most crucial? This is not typically a sign of AD, just a sign of interpersonal communication dysfunction. This is "selective memory loss." However, we also are unable to remember things that are definitely in our memory banks. How many times were we unable to answer questions on tests even though we studied, and then recalled the answer as soon as the paper was turned in? How often do we forget a name, just as we need it, but then remember it 30 seconds later? These are failures of memory retrieval, and also vary with concentration, mood, stress, and a large number of other conditions.

In PD, memory problems are sometimes seen as worse than they are because some PD patients become slow thinking (bradyphrenia) or are impaired by their medications. In the case of bradyphrenia, the patients are frequently not given sufficient time to answer questions or solve problems, and are assumed to not understand, when they simply haven't been given enough time.

DEMENTIA TESTING

There are several different tests that may be performed to determine if a patient is actually demented or not. Sometimes the patient may have "MCI" (mild cognitive impairment), "pseudo-dementia" or a psychiatric problem that interferes with normal thinking. Sometimes "formal testing," that is, sophisticated testing by a PhD neuropsychologist, is performed to obtain very detailed and validated testing, both to determine if there is a problem and what the depth of the problem is. This testing also identifies strengths that can be utilized to compensate for intellectual or memory weaknesses.

The most commonly administered test in the office is the mini–mental state exam (MMSE), so-called because it is very brief. It is a 30-point questionnaire that tests, in a very quick and superficial manner, orientation (where are we; what is today's date; what is the season; etc.), memory (recall three objects), "working memory" (spell a word forwards and then backwards, or perform serial subtractions), and language and construction (name objects, write a sentence, and copy a picture).

The generally accepted definition of dementia is a decline in memory and cognition that causes a decline in social function. Some people lead such structured lives, doing the same thing each and everyday at the same time, that dementia doesn't appear until the patient's memory and cognition are quite impaired, whereas a university professor or a lawyer might experience difficulties at the very earliest stages of the condition.

MEMORY

The memory failure in PD is different from the memory problems in AD. In AD there is no memory trace. The memory bank is blank. The PD patient initially lays down a memory trace but may not be able to recall a memory, but, if given some cues, often can. In other words, the memory itself exists, but access to the memory is faulty. So, for example, in the standard office examination for dementia, the MMSE is given. The easier memory questions ask the person to memorize three words. As soon as the words are spoken, the patient is asked to recall them in order to make sure that they were heard correctly, as well as to determine how many times the person needs to hear the words in order to remember them. A normal person hears the words once and remembers them. An AD patient may need to hear the words a few times before committing them to memory. A minute or so later the person is asked to recall the words. A normal person recalls all three, sometimes just two, whereas a demented person may not recall any, or just one. The AD patient may not even recall being asked to do this task, whereas the PD patient will usually say, "I know you gave me three words, but I just can't remember them." The AD patient may be given some cues but these don't help. He may make up answers, whereas the PD patient will often benefit from cues. If the word is "baseball," for example, then giving the hint, "It's a sport," may provide the spark of recognition that triggers the answer, whereas the AD patient is unlikely to benefit from these hints.

All patients with memory problems may recall things incorrectly, but the PD patient is much less likely to "confabulate," that is, to make things up out of whole cloth. The PD patient is more likely to say, "I don't know," rather than creating an answer that makes sense to the patient, if not to anyone else.

Memory, in all disorders, is affected in a retrograde (backwards) manner. This means that the more recent memories are affected more than older memories. This does not mean that only recent memories are affected. Older memories may be impaired as well, but the problem is primarily centered on recent things. This means, of course, that learning becomes seriously impaired. Learning requires memory. Once the ability to retain new memories is reduced, then the ability to learn is disrupted as well.

Because the older memories are more secure, family members are often fooled into thinking the patient is "sharp as a tack" because he remembers the menu for his wedding 50 years ago. Unfortunately, while his memory for the wedding may be accurate, he cannot recall if he just ate breakfast, lunch, or supper.

INSIGHT

Many people with memory and thinking problems lose insight into their problems. This is perhaps the biggest problem for demented people. Most people have a pretty good idea of their limitations. If a person has a complicated schedule he writes the appointments down and uses a calendar or a smartphone. Many doctors carry index cards to keep track of their hospitalized patients, appointments, telephone numbers, and a variety of other things because they *know* they cannot possibly remember them all. Some of us rely more on our memories than others, but we all take notes to some extent, and people who know their memories are not completely reliable will take extra steps to compensate. The demented patient usually cannot be trained to do this. In addition, when we are asked to recall some bit of information and our memory doesn't jibe with reality, we usually deduce that our memory failed us.

If I recall that my son was to meet me at 2 p.m. in a certain location and he doesn't show up then, I'll either deduce that he's late or that I got the time or location wrong. A demented person may not make that deduction and therefore not take steps to counter the missed appointment. If I recall that a ballgame is on TV at a particular time and I then cannot find it, I'll check the TV listings to confirm my memory. Demented people don't do this. They either ignore the mismatch, or sometimes insist that they are correct and everyone else is wrong. Instead of, "I must have gotten the time wrong," it becomes, "The darned newspaper screwed up the time," "The TV changed the time," and so on. This can lead to serious arguments in the home, when the demented person insists that his recall of events is correct, despite an ever-lengthening history of worsened memory function.

An 80-year-old retired engineer insists that his grandchildren are visiting later that day, although both work full-time in other states. He yells at his wife to try to force her to bake special cookies for them. When she tells him that she spoke with them earlier in the week, and that they aren't coming, he tells her that she's lying.

A 73-year-old woman knows her memory is failing her. She sometimes calls her daughter every five minutes to ask if she's on her way over. She keeps forgetting that she just called, but she's so afraid of forgetting anything that she feels compelled to call.

Sometimes, inaccurate or incorrect information gets incorporated into the memory bank. This happens to everyone. A standard experiment in psychology is to stage an incident that is completely unexpected to the class, then to ask the students to reconstruct the event. Typically the recollections are quite different. Certain events are remembered accurately while others are not, or possibly weren't observed, and the person's imagination weaves the observed actions together in a memory that makes sense and has internal consistency. However, the "filled-in" events may not actually have occurred so that the recollection is not at all accurate. In the case of the demented person, dreams, TV or newspaper stories, or anecdotes about family and friends may get incorporated into new memories. Thus, incorrect memories get stored among the "real" memories.

A *73-year-old woman with PD decides to withdraw all her money from a bank because she saw a TV show on the Great Depression. Thinking that this is current news but noticing that no one around her is panicking, she believes that she has an insight that others haven't understood yet, so she can withdraw her money in time to prevent calamity.*

THINKING PROBLEMS

Memory is only one of the problems people with dementia have. They are unable to solve simple problems such as negotiating their way out of a house they can't recall having been in before. They can't figure out, perhaps, how the water tap works, particularly if it's unlike something they've seen before. For example, it can be a trial for a demented person to figure out how the heat-sensitive devices in the bathrooms of airports work. For many of us it may have been a challenge the first time as well, but we either figured it out or watched others for hints on how to solve the problem of getting the water faucet to run or the toilet to flush. For a demented person, figuring out what to do, or even how to copy how others do the chore is impossible. Unwrapping certain packages can be difficult, or figuring out how to insert batteries, or even that batteries are required. Everyday chores that we all take for granted without batting an eyelash may be major confrontations for a demented person.

DIFFERENTIAL DIAGNOSIS

There are several reasons for PD patients to develop memory problems. The most important are those that are reversible. Anticholinergic drugs—which have the chemical property of interfering with the neurotransmitter acetylcholine—are commonly used to treat an overactive bladder, and also to treat tremor or drooling in PD. As a side effect they often worsen memory, and can produce Alzheimer's-like problems. Many of the drugs that work in the brain may produce various levels of confusion, and may, in an older person, produce an Alzheimer's picture.

Infections of various sorts may make the patient delirious and therefore appear to be demented. Thyroid disease also can do this, but is very rare.

Unfortunately, most of the causes of memory problems are not reversible. These are the dementia syndromes. People with PD may become demented from PD itself, but other problems, such as strokes, AD, and dementia with Lewy bodies (DLB) may also occur.

ALZHEIMER'S DISEASE

AD is the most common disorder causing dementia in the Western world (in Africa, more people have AIDS-related dementia and getting to old age is uncommon). Unfortunately, in this case lightning *can* strike twice. Having one bad neurological disease does not protect someone from developing a second. In fact, it appears that having PD may put the patient at increased risk for developing AD. Behavioral problems and impaired judgment are the norm. One of the main problems is the patient's lack of insight into the problem.

STROKES

A stroke is a "cerebrovascular accident." Most commonly, strokes are caused by blockages of blood flow to a portion of the brain. As a result this part of the brain dies. Typically the event causes the sudden onset of a new neurological problem, almost always weakness, numbness, or clumsiness of one side of the body. Single strokes do not cause dementia, but accumulated strokes may. The classic story for this type of dementia is "stepwise progression" of the dementia. The patient suddenly becomes more confused, and then either stabilizes at that level or even improves a bit, until another stroke occurs, leaving the person suddenly worse yet again. This generally occurs in people who have the stroke risk factors of high blood pressure, heart disease, and diabetes, and have had the usual type of stroke that causes one-sided weakness, or loss of vision to one side, or a sudden problem with language. Tiny strokes that would generally not cause any new problem in a healthy, mentally intact person, may cause significant neurological declines in people who are already mildly demented. Generally, a magnetic resonance imaging (MRI) of the brain will show that the patient has had multiple tiny strokes, even though the patient and family are unaware of any stroke-like event.

In addition to frank strokes, patients often have "small vessel ischemic disease" (SVID), which is an MRI term, also called "leukoaraiosis" (weakening of the white matter) on computerized tomography (CT) scans. This describes a pathological change in the white matter of the brain, which is believed to be due to years of slowly developing blood vessel narrowing and hardening. This causes harm to the parts of the brain cells that convey messages from one part of the brain to another. Because everything in the brain is connected to almost every other part of the brain, this causes major problems. These problems develop slowly, however, so that the patient undergoes a slow, but continuous decline in memory and cognition primarily. These changes also contribute though to the motor problems in PD, exacerbating the slowness, stiffness, balance and posture problems as well as the mental impairments. These brain changes are associated with strokes, as well as the major risk factors for strokes, namely, high blood pressure, diabetes and heart disease of all types.

DEMENTIA WITH LEWY BODIES

DLB is an increasingly recognized disorder with an interesting and illustrative history. The "Lewy body" is a pathological sphere that is seen under the microscope in people with PD. It's been recognized as an important pathological feature of the disease since the 1930s, but has only been considered a microscopic requirement for the disease in the past 20 years or so. The name of the disorder is based on the pathology that is seen in the brain autopsy. So, this is a dementia in which Lewy bodies are seen on stained sections of the brain when viewed under a microscope.

I personally do not like this name. For a time it was called Lewy body dementia or diffuse Lewy body disease. I prefer the last name, as I find it difficult telling a patient that the name of their disease is "dementia." We even know Alzheimer's dementia as "Alzheimer's disease" these days, so why not Lewy body disease? In the early 1960s a group of neuropathologists reported the first case of this disorder, in a patient who had died in a chronic care institution, with advanced dementia. In PD the Lewy bodies are seen primarily in a small region in the brainstem, the part of the brain that connects with the spinal cord. There are a few Lewy bodies also seen in other brainstem and lower sites, but in this case the Lewy bodies were seen over the cortex, the outer mantle of the brain, in profusion.

Over the next few decades a handful of other cases were also described, but very rarely. Then, all of a sudden, a report from England stated that DLB was the second most common cause of dementia in England, after being considered an extraordinarily rare disease throughout the world. How could this be? Basically advances in cell staining techniques by pathologists allowed more and more Lewy bodies to be seen, and with these new techniques, and a greater interest in finding these abnormalities, many more cases were found. It is unclear if DLB is the second or third most common cause of dementia in the United States, but it is clearly a lot more common than had been thought. Many doctors are very unfamiliar with this and often mistake the condition for AD.

Among neurologists and geriatric psychiatrists, there is a lot of debate as to whether DLB and PD are the same condition or different ones with a degree of overlap. They are very similar. We use the term DLB if the dementia began before or shortly after the motor features of PD. DLB patients often have marked changes in the level of their confusion during each day and may also have periods of being unresponsive, looking like they're asleep with their eyes open.

EVALUATION OF PD PATIENTS WITH DEMENTIA

How PD patients with dementia should be evaluated is a contentious issue. I think that virtually all neurologists would agree that the reversible causes for dementia should be investigated. A blood clot on the brain sustained during a fall can be an explanation. A rare patient with thyroid dysfunction, low vitamin B_{12} or folic acid, or neurosyphillis may be detected, but, quite frankly, I'm not sure I've come across any in over three decades in the field. The real issues have to do with whether the patient has PD, DLB, AD, or MID (multi-infarct dementia). Because none of these are treatable, in the sense that we have no special interventions to slow the progression of any of them, and the symptomatic treatments are identical, depending only on the symptoms, not the disease process itself, it is unclear to me that testing is of much value. I will frequently order neuropsychological tests, but these are primarily to identify how impaired a patient is, something that a family will often not recognize, how well preserved another area of thinking may be, and perhaps most importantly, to help develop a strategy for coping with current problems and anticipating future problems. Safety is always an issue.

There is little value in my opinion in obtaining brain imaging. It is true that this may be considered the "standard of care" in many American communities, but as far as I'm concerned the MRI rarely helps with management of the patient. Yes, it is true, that the MRI may make the diagnosis of the dementia more accurate, although not always. AD cannot be diagnosed on the MRI, nor can DLB. Only strokes and SVID can be seen on MRI, or brain tumors and blood clots pressing on the brain. While these latter may occur in people with PD, they are very uncommon, and when they do occur, they usually cause "focal signs," that is, evidence of malfunction of a particular part of the brain, rather than global dysfunction as occurs with the other dementing disorders. Some patients or families consider it incumbent on their doctors to order every test in the book. Some doctors feel the same thing: If they're the specialist, they should order lots of tests. Other doctors worry that if they don't order a test and something bad happens they will be legally at risk, even if they themselves don't believe the test will provide any help in caring for the patient.

TREATMENT

There have been very few studies of the treatment of dementia in PD. Only one drug, rivastigmine (Exelon), has been approved by the Food and Drug Administration (FDA) for this. As of the second edition of this book, a single large, well-designed and well-executed study has been published. Aside from this there have been small studies involving handfuls of patients and therefore these have been less reliable than a large multicenter trial. Three of the four drugs used in AD are from the same chemical family called cholinesterase inhibitors (CEI). These drugs act to inhibit, or block, an enzyme that breaks down acetylcholine, a chemical found normally in the brain that is thought to be important in memory. One of the reasons that scientists looked at the possible role of acetylcholine in memory is that anticholinergics, drugs that block the action of acetylcholine, often caused patients to suffer memory problems. Interestingly, the main role of anticholinergic drugs used to be PD! These drugs are still used, but not very much. They are particularly useful in treating tremor but also to reduce bladder activity and drooling. Unfortunately, in addition to sometimes causing memory loss, confusion, and hallucinations, these drugs also cause constipation.

It turns out that in AD there is a reduced amount of acetylcholine so the notion that this chemical is involved in memory was reinforced. Three drugs—donepezil, galantamine, and rivastigmine—have all been shown to improve thinking, attention, and mood in people with AD. Studies of the brains of PD patients with dementia have shown that there is an even greater reduction of acetylcholine than there is in AD. This suggests that the potential benefits might be even greater. On the other hand, the fact that drugs that block acetylcholine help PD motor symptoms suggests that drugs that do the opposite may worsen the motor aspects of PD, particularly tremor. There was therefore a "clinical equipoise" about using the drugs in PD. There were hopes about benefits and concerns about side effects and these have mostly balanced out. Some studies, however, have been performed.

The three CEIs used for AD, donepezil (Aricept), galantamine (Reminyl), and rivastigmine (Exelon) actually have very little effect on average. Interestingly, although the drugs were theoretically developed to improve memory, they have only a small effect on memory. The main benefits of the drugs are in attention, mood, interest, and hallucinations. There is generally less benefit in memory and thinking.

In the single large study of one of these drugs in PD patients with dementia, which involved over 500 subjects, rivastigmine was found to be helpful for the dementia and well tolerated. Only a small number of patients suffered worsening of the motor symptoms of PD; however, there were some. The benefits of the drug, however, were modest. In terms of cognition, "Clinically meaningful improvement was observed in 19.8% of patients in the rivastigmine group and 14.5% of those in the placebo group." This means that out of every 100 patients with PD only 5 will benefit more than if they took a sugar pill.

On the other hand, if we look at worsening, about 9% more patients receiving the placebo got worse over the 24 weeks of the study than those on the rivastigmine. The study report concluded, "The absolute differences in the rates of improvement (between subjects taking rivastigmine and placebo) were small, and the majority of patients who were treated with rivastigmine (80.2%) had no clinically meaningful improvement" as measured by scales used for cognition and memory.

There have been several small studies involving all of the CEI drugs in PD, and all have shown pretty much the same outcome. The drugs have modest benefits, but only in a minority of patients. The drugs are generally well tolerated but some PD patients do suffer worsening of tremor and rigidity. Long-term data are not available yet.

A fourth drug for AD has not yet been tested adequately in PD patients. Its generic name is memantine (Namenda), and it appears to have similar efficacy to the CEI drugs. It is a chemical relative of amantadine, which is a drug used to treat the motor symptoms of PD, so it is possible that this drug will have special benefits in PD patients. So far, the little data published suggests that this is not true.

In short, there is only one drug currently approved for the treatment of dementia in PD—rivastibmine (Exelon). The other similar drugs probably work as well but have not been adequately tested. These drugs help some people considerably, but not most.

DISEASE PROGRESSION

When dementia occurs in PD it is part of the illness, and, like all neurodegenerative disorders, always progresses. The decline over time has been measured, and, like other aspects of PD, progresses at its own rate in each individual. Dementia is frequently accompanied by apathy, which is protective. The patient doesn't care.

8

. . . .

Hallucinations

Hallucinations occur in about 30% of Parkinson's disease (PD) patients taking medications for their condition. PD itself does not cause hallucinations. The problem is almost always from medication, usually the PD medications. Very often the hallucinations begin after a new medication is added or an old one is increased, but they may occur without any recent medicine changes. Even if one new medication precipitates the hallucinations, that one medication is not necessarily the problem. It is the accumulated effects of all the medications working on the brain. It's like getting drunk. The last drink puts you over the top. Hallucinations generally don't cause problems, but they may.

Visual hallucinations occur in about 30% of PD patients taking PD medications. This has been confirmed in a few studies in different PD centers around the world. Few doctors are aware that this side effect is so common and therefore don't ask about it. In most cases the hallucinations are recognized as unreal by the patient and are tolerated as a somewhat annoying or even amusing side effect, but the hallucinations can be scary, either because they appear threatening or because the very idea of a hallucination is a threat to one's sanity.

It may be thought to be the opening salvo in Alzheimer's disease (AD) or another condition in which one starts to "lose one's mind."

A new medication is begun and after a few days the PD patient starts seeing children outdoors playing in the tree, and raises a concern that the children are unsupervised and might injure themselves. No one else sees these children. Every two or three days the same vision occurs, and, after a while the patient just keeps this to himself so others won't think he's "crazy."

A patient has been taking Levodopa (Sinemet) for several years, and without any medication change she starts to see two strange adults wearing "funny costumes" sitting on the sofa looking at her. When she talks to them they ignore her. This bothers her so she gets up from her chair to confront one of these people and as she approaches them they suddenly disappear.

There is often confusion about what a hallucination is, and how it differs from other peculiar false sensations. A hallucination is a perception that occurs without any stimulus. When one sees things, while awake, that are not really there, we call these visual hallucinations. We have all had auditory hallucinations, hearing a voice or a sound that no one else heard. We hear our children or spouse calling our name, but the house is empty, or the spouse denies making a sound. But we don't hear these too often and they are usually single sounds, like our name, and not complex sentences. In PD, hallucinations occur as a result of the medications we use for treating motor problems. PD itself does not cause hallucinations* so that if we stop the medications the hallucinations go away. Typically the PD patient sees things rather

---

*DLB does cause visual hallucinations even when the patient is not taking any medications.

than hearing, smelling, tasting, or feeling things, although these may happen as well.

Hallucinations in PD are very different from hallucinations that occur in psychiatric disorders such as schizophrenia, in which patients usually have auditory hallucinations. They hear things that others don't. These are usually voices, although other sounds may be heard as well, and these voices often say nasty things about the patient. When the patient feels that he is a foul person who others hate, the voices will confirm this, telling the patient that he does smell bad, that everyone does despise him, and that he should hide away from other people because they hate him. But when the patient thinks that he is an emissary from God, he will hear words from God, or voices telling him how wonderful and holy he is.

In PD, auditory hallucinations are much less common, and when they do occur they usually occur in people who already are having visual hallucinations. The most striking difference between the hallucinations in PD and those occurring in psychiatric disorders is that the PD patient's hallucinations are usually relatively free of emotional content. In schizophrenia the hallucinations almost always have major emotional associations that fit in with the peculiar beliefs the patient has during this psychotic period. The PD patient sees children in ballet costumes, women in dressing gowns, circus dogs, construction crews digging up their yard. They may hear party sounds coming from another room in the house, or people talking outside the room though the actual words are indistinct. Even when the hallucination should cause a stir in emotions, this frequently doesn't happen. For example, a woman sees her husband, dead for ten years, lying in bed next to her, but she is neither happy to see him nor sentimental. "How should I feel? It's a hallucination. He's been dead for ten years."

The hallucinations with PD medications are closer to the hallucinations seen on lysergic acid diethylamide (LSD) or other "psychedelic" drugs, and for good reason. The drugs that treat PD are chemically related to these psychedelic drugs and therefore share some of the same properties.

Hallucinations in PD are extremely interesting. They are fairly similar among different individuals. Usually they occur in people who are otherwise not mentally engaged. They occur at home, while the patient is reading a magazine or watching TV, usually alone. While the hallucinations more commonly occur at night, they may occur in the daytime as well. Some people see their hallucinations only in the shadows, while others see them only in the light. One of my patients saw small red crabs under the night-light but not in the darker parts of the room. The hallucinations tend to be the same each time. One patient saw three girls wearing ballet costumes dancing in the driveway when she washed the dinner dishes. She never had other types of hallucinations, and the three girls were always the same and always dressed the same. Sometimes patients see inanimate objects such as statues. One of my patients told me he was hallucinating. Since strange things sometimes occur in the hospital I asked him how he knew what he saw wasn't real. He told me he saw a tractor outside the window and since he was on the fourth floor of the hospital he knew it couldn't be real.

The occurrence of hallucinations is to a large extent determined by the environment. In a low-stimulus setting they are more likely. In an interesting research study, PD patients who had visual hallucinations on L-Dopa at home were brought into the hospital to be studied while hallucinating. They were given L-Dopa by intravenous infusion at a much higher dose than they had received at home, yet not a single patient hallucinated, although they all had been having hallucinations every night at home. Somehow, the novelty of the hospital setting kept them from developing hallucinations. The more activity there is in the environment, the less likely it is for hallucinations to appear.

Sometimes the hallucinated people interact among themselves. They gesticulate and appear to be talking to each other although no sounds can be heard by the patient. The hallucinations may get angry with each other and storm out of the room, slamming the door, but without making any sound. Usually the hallucinations ignore the patient, even when he talks or gestures to them. Sometimes the hallucinations will talk to the patient, in which case the patient may carry on a conversation.

Most PD patients have insight into their hallucinations and recognize that the hallucinations aren't real. In fact, many patients will not share their hallucinations with their family for fear of having them think they're either "crazy" or have developed AD. Hallucinations are actually uncommon in AD.

When the patient loses insight, that is, believes the hallucinations are real, the problems usually begin. A patient may set an extra place at the dinner table for the "guest." A bowl of water may be placed on the floor for the "dog" that lives under the bed. Or, more problematically, the police may be called to get rid of the strange man standing in the kitchen.

Sometimes the hallucinations are tiny, such as ants or other bugs, but sometimes they are of smaller–than–life-size people. These are called "Lilliputian," after the small world in *Gulliver's Travels*, but it is unknown if the size has any significance. I am unaware of any reports of larger-than-life hallucinations.

A *60-year-old woman sees little people living in her houseplant. She believes they are "up to no good," so she spends her day keeping an eye on them to prevent mischief.*

Almost half the patients with visual hallucinations also have auditory hallucinations. The auditory hallucinations tend to be less distinct than the visual. Whereas the visual hallucinations are seen clearly, the auditory hallucinations tend to be less clear, such as music coming from outdoors, crowd noises, conversations from a distance with the words indistinct. Tactile hallucinations, such as feeling things that aren't really there, as well as smell and taste hallucinations, are much less common.

A 75-year-old man with PD reports "critters" that crawl on his skin every night as soon as he gets into bed. No matter how hard he looks for them he can't see them and he can't catch them. He knows they're not real because he rolls over on them yet he never crushes them to find a dead "critter." They are mildly uncomfortable but not painful. Sometimes he sees them under his shirt but when he points this out his family tells him they are not real. He has tried getting rid of them by showering, drying himself and then running out of the bathroom naked, slamming the door behind them, to keep them locked in the bathroom, but nevertheless they are still on his skin when he puts his pyjamas on. While he "knows" they are not real, they still feel as if they are completely real. Antipsychotic medication reduces their presence but does not eliminate them.

DIFFERENTIAL DIAGNOSIS OF HALLUCINATIONS

It is not always clear when a patient is hallucinating. Some people confuse realistic or "vivid" dreams with hallucinations. But such dreams are one of the side effects of L-Dopa and some other PD medications. PD patients will discuss things that they dreamed about the previous night as if they actually occurred. Family members will deduce that the person has been hallucinating. In actuality, there is a large difference between objects or people seen when awake and alert and those appearing in a dream. The implications and treatments are different.

Another common source of confusion is illusions. An illusion is a misperception, such as seeing a bear in a shadow, and these can be common, especially in people who have visual or hearing impairments. Deaf people very commonly mishear and answer questions quite different from the ones they were asked. Illusions are not considered "problems" until they become common enough to undermine the person's interpretation of the environment. Visual illusions may be due to the PD medications. Auditory illusions are not considered to be medication related. Of course, there may be a PD patient or two who experiences PD medication–induced auditory illusions, but this must be considered quite rare. Drug-induced visual illusions may possibly be a problem that develops before frank visual hallucinations.

It is well known that PD patients have a multitude of sleep problems (see Chapter 12). Sometimes they begin to dream slightly before they fall asleep, so they may seem to be hallucinating, as their eyes are open. This also may occur as they are awakening.

Some people with PD become "confused." This term means many different things to different people, but usually the family will use this to mean both disorientation and misidentification of things or people around them. When people act in a confused manner, such as thinking that their spouse has been replaced by an impostor, that they are not at home although they really are at home, the family may believe this too represents hallucinations, that the person is seeing unusual things. Doctors believe that this confusional spell is a form of delirium, in which the memory of common things is distorted, so that some objects at home are familiar but some look strange or out of place. This lends an air of a horror movie, so that the poor patient becomes agitated, as if some force is "playing games" with his sanity. This, of course, makes the whole situation much worse since anxiety, or nervousness, is the opposite of what is needed, namely, calmness.

And, finally, not all visual hallucinations are due to the PD medications! There is a syndrome called "Bonnet's syndrome" after the doctor who described his elderly father starting to have visual hallucinations as he lost his vision. Elderly people, without any problems with their memory or thinking, and without PD, may start to see things as they become blind. Interestingly, since the hallucinations are generated by the brain and not the eyes, and all the patients have visual problems, the hallucinations tend to be seen far more clearly than could be seen in real life.

A 76-year-old woman with severely impaired eyesight in both eyes has a cataract removed from her better eye. After surgery she suffers a complication, making the better eye now the worse eye. Several hours after this deterioration of her vision she sees a large spider in her kitchen. Because she's alone she leaves her house to get a neighbor's help since she is phobic of spiders. The neighbor isn't home and when the patient returns to her house the door is covered by large spiders. She can't see well enough to venture far from her house so she waits outside for her daughter to return. While she's standing, a gang of motorcycle riders is pulled off the road by a policeman and made to park on her lawn. Every time she tries to signal the policeman he turns aside, so he never sees her signaling. The crowd and the motorcycles make no noise. When her daughter returns, she is taken to the emergency department (ED) of the local hospital where she is given an antipsychotic drug, despite no history of any psychiatric or thinking problem, and referred to the psychiatrist who then calls me. The patient tells me that the hospital experience is peculiar because the ED is decorated with brightly colored parrots sitting on perches in the corridor. She finds this bizarre but a welcome decorating touch. Aside from her severely impaired vision she is normal. She is reassured and a few weeks later the hallucinations resolve completely. She suffers from Bonnet's syndrome. She does not have PD or take any PD medications.

Thus, although the most likely explanation for visual hallucinations is a PD drug, it may be due to something else.

Who experiences hallucinations? Anyone taking PD medications. However, there have been a few "risk factors" identified, that is, conditions that put some people at greater risk than others for developing hallucinations. Aside from the medications, and some are more likely to produce this problem than others, the most important predisposing factor is dementia. People with memory or cognitive problems are at much higher risk for this type of side effect than are people whose memory and thinking are normal. The various PD medications have never been compared head-to-head for side effects; however, the dopamine agonists, bromocriptine (Parlodel), rotigotine (Neupro), pramipexole (Mirapex), and ropinerole (Requip) have been compared to L-Dopa, and all are more likely to cause hallucinations than L-Dopa. It is likely that anticholinergic drugs such as benztropine (Cogentin) and trihexiphenidyl (Artane) do as well. How amantadine (Symmetrel) compares to L-Dopa in terms of hallucination potential is unknown.

Although this condition is different from Bonnet's syndrome, there are data showing that there is a mildly increased risk of visual hallucinations in PD patients with diminished vision. However, this association is mostly statistical and does not hold up for individual cases.

TREATMENT OF HALLUCINATIONS

Not all hallucinations need to be treated. In fact, most do not. What is most important is reassurance. Once the patient and family learn that 30% of PD patients who take medication for their PD have hallucinations and that the hallucinations are medication side effects, "tricks" of the mind, then their worries are usually reduced. Some patients actually enjoy their hallucinations!

A *78-year-old man does not report hallucinations but when asked if he hallucinates he admits that he sees a baby every night when he goes to bed. He smiles as he says this, then comments, "He's so good. He never makes a sound."*

On the other hand, some patients do not enjoy having strangers appear suddenly in their living room watching them as they watch TV. And although most visual hallucinations are not threatening, some are.

A 60-year-old man reports having visual hallucinations. He sees people outside his den. "How do you know they're hallucinations if they're outside?" I ask. "Well, every morning I see a group of nuns wearing habits who start building me a deck."

A 68-year-old woman also reports seeing nuns wearing habits, but they are not building a deck. They have fangs that drip blood.

Obviously, seeing a nun with fangs dripping blood is not a pleasant experience. Scary or unpleasant hallucinations should not be tolerated and should be treated, when possible. It is also important to treat hallucinations when the patient acts as if the hallucination is real—setting extra places at the dinner table, calling the police, putting out clothing, and so on. The decision to treat or not treat is then based on the effect the hallucinations have on the patient.

An 80-year-old man started seeing snakes crawling into his house when he opened the front door although he was in a large New England city. In the house itself he frequently saw large rats that he would try to hit with a club. He purchased several very strong rat traps which he put around the house. His wife was concerned he would break his hand in the traps because they were so strong. He only partially believed his wife about the rats being hallucinated. He thought that some might not be real but that some definitely were, so he was angry that she removed the rat traps.

A patient driving down a street in her neighborhood is stunned to see a tyrannosaurus picking up a car. She swerves to avoid hitting the dinosaur and is picked up by a policeman who wonders if she is drunk.

A patient driving a car is bothered by three small people in the back seat of his car. He is very unsure of what to do. On the one hand he wants them out of the car, but on the other, he knows they're not real and that if he stops his car to get them out, he might be picked up by a policeman and taken to the hospital.

TREATMENT

The family and caregivers should tell the patient in a matter-of-fact tone that the hallucinations are "tricks" of the mind, side effects of the PD medications, that the patient is not losing his mind. It is best not to humor the patient by agreeing that the stranger is well dressed, or is tall. It is best to be truthful but also understanding and supportive. "Yes, I know that this thing you're seeing looks as real as I do, but it's not. I do not see it, and you know the doctor told you that the medications you take can cause visual hallucinations." If possible the patient should then be "redirected," that is, forced to focus on another topic.

The next step in dealing with the hallucinations is to try to reduce the PD medications and any other medications that act on the brain. Mental side effects are often due to the combined effects of drugs. Because hallucinations are generated by the brain, only drugs that enter the brain are possible culprits. Many drugs do not get into the brain so the side effects they cause do not include behavior problems. In many cases the hallucinations begin shortly after one medication is increased or a new medication is started; however, the hallucinations aren't necessarily due directly to the one drug change, but rather to the combined effects of all the brain-active medications. The situation is very much like getting drunk. While a person may get drunk after their second martini, this occurs only because of the three whiskey sours and the two cans of beer that preceded it. Just as the alcohol level increased with each drink, the PD medication effects often represent the effects of the L-Dopa plus the selegiline plus the antianxiety medication and the sleeping medication.

When medications are reduced to the lowest level that can be tolerated without a significant reduction in mobility, then they can't be reduced any further. At this point there are two options for further treatment. In the United States virtually all PD specialists would add quetiapine (Seroquel), an antipsychotic drug, as it combats hallucinations (and delusions; see Chapter 9) and does not worsen mobility. In England one of the cholinesterase inhibitors (AD medications) would be used if the situation was not an emergency. Quetiapine, like other antipsychotic drugs, is used primarily to treat schizophrenia. While this condition is quite different from schizophrenia, hallucinations are part of both, and it turns out that the drugs that treat the hallucinations of schizophrenia are usually helpful in treating the hallucinations in PD. The main issue, however, has to do with the side effects of these drugs. All of the old drugs used to treat schizophrenia cause the patients to look as if they have PD. If the patients have PD to begin with, then these medications make their motor function considerably worse. Obviously, these drugs are not useful.

Since 1991, however, newer drugs have been developed that are much less likely to cause people to look as if they have PD, and two of these have been found to be well tolerated by patients with PD. Unfortunately, the other drugs are not so well tolerated and often worsen mobility or tremor. The two drugs that work in PD without causing worsened motor function are clozapine and quetiapine.

Clozapine has been the subject of two independent, high-quality studies that proved that the drug was helpful, well tolerated, and relatively safe. Unfortunately clozapine can lower the white blood cell count in about 1% to 2% of older people, so the Food and Drug Administration requires weekly blood counts for the first six months followed by blood counts every other week for the next six months, then monthly tests thereafter. In Europe, patients are required to have their blood tested only once each month after the first six months. Clozapine is the most effective antipsychotic drug in the world, but because of the white blood cell problem, and some other problems that occur in doses much higher than are used in PD, it is rarely used outside of PD.

Quetiapine has become the drug of choice for treating hallucinations because, like clozapine, it does not worsen motor function. It appears, however, to be less effective so that higher doses of it are needed compared with clozapine. In fact, although most PD experts think quetiapine is useful, the few studies that have been reported found that it was well tolerated in terms of not making motor problems worse, but it didn't actually help the psychosis. Nevertheless, the American Academy of Neurology's task force on PD recommended "considering" quetiapine for treating hallucinations, along with clozapine. Quetiapine, like all antipsychotic drugs, is associated with an unexplained increase in the death rate of older people.

We therefore recommend reducing PD medications first, then introducing quetiapine starting with 12.5 mg at bedtime. Quetiapine is a very sedating medication. Quetiapine also causes orthostatic hypotension, a condition in which patients' blood pressure drops when they stand up.

There are data to suggest that all of the other antipsychotic drugs—risperidone, olanzapine, and aripiprazole, for example—are not good drugs to use in people with PD because of their side effect of increasing motor dysfunction. However, sometimes these antipsychotic drugs may work well for some PD patients without making motor function worse. If something is helpful and well tolerated, it shouldn't be stopped because the drug is not tolerated by others.

In general, a low dose of quetiapine is begun, usually 12.5 mg, given at bedtime, then increased as needed depending on the response. If there is no response at all, either for the hallucinations or in terms of increased sedation, then the dose may be increased, even as soon as the second night. If the patient is sedated by the medication, then the increase should occur more slowly. The dose should be increased until the bothersome behavior is no longer bothersome. Keep in mind that it is best to aim for the lowest dose of quetiapine that allows the patient to be comfortable. It is not necessary to completely get rid of the hallucinations, just to get them "under control," so that they don't upset the patient.

Occasionally the hallucinations bother the caregiver more than they bother the patient. Spouses may see the hallucinations as a sign that their loved one is losing his or her mind and may find the sight of their husband or wife hallucinating intolerable. In such cases it is important for everyone to remember who the sick person is and who and why medications are being given. It is usually not a good idea to treat one person in order to make the other one feel more comfortable. Of course, this does need to be done sometimes, but it should always be clear who is being treated and for what reason.

An older method of treating the hallucinations was to take the patient off all PD medications for one to two weeks and then restart them at much lower doses. This was called a "drug holiday" and was in vogue in the late 1970s. Unfortunately this treatment was unsafe and in the long run did not work.

Patients who develop hallucinations tend to continue having them unless their medications are reduced. Therefore, once the anti-psychotic drug is begun, it usually has to remain in place unless the PD medications are altered.

A 76-year-old man complains that each afternoon the same man appears, standing in front of his television, blocking the view. While the patient doesn't feel threatened, and wouldn't mind tolerating the hallucination if it just stood to the side, blocking the TV is not acceptable, so he wants treatment.

A 70-year-old man had been hospitalized for psychotic symptoms, seeing people and for delusions, thinking his wife had been seeing other men. He reported that when he walked outside, one of his wife's lovers would spray him with cologne so that they'd be able to smell him in advance of his being seen. He was successfully treated but on returning to the office he was having auditory hallucinations, which were getting worse. He stopped taking his antipsychotic medication because he heard the voice of his psychiatrist telling him to stop taking the medication he, himself, had prescribed.

A question I frequently encounter is, why should the hallucinations develop in someone whose medications haven't changed in a year or more? The answer is that although the medication isn't changing, the brain is. With age our brains shrink, just like almost everything else. With advancing PD and a general shrinkage of the brain, the brain becomes more sensitive to medication side effects.

Delusions

The drug treatment of Parkinson's disease (PD) causes false and irrational beliefs, usually paranoid, in about 5% to 10% of patients. Most commonly, patients think their spouse is cheating on them, but they may also think people are spying, tapping the phone, stealing money, planning to burglarize the house, and so on. This problem is extremely bothersome to all involved. It is usually treatable.

Psychosis used to be defined as a major mental illness characterized by the loss of mental and social functioning due to impaired reality testing. The definition excluded people who were delirious or drunk. In other words, psychotic people were normal in terms of their memory, problem-solving skills, and attention span, but misinterpreted what was going on around them. Their "reality" was different from everyone else's. The current definition of psychosis I find less clear. A person is said to be psychotic if he suffers from one or more of the following: delusions, hallucinations, disorganized thinking or speech, or grossly disorganized or catatonic behavior. For the PD patient, psychotic behavior translates into delusions and hallucinations.

The topic of hallucinations is covered in Chapter 8. PD patients do not develop disorganized thinking or abnormal speech.

Delusions are false or irrational beliefs. These beliefs are sometimes based on a markedly abnormal interpretation of an event or statement, or, more commonly, based on no evidence at all. The irrationality of the belief and the irrationality of the patient make logical arguments against the delusion a wasted effort.

A 30-year-old man believes Al Qaeda agents are following him because he saw a man with a beard who looked like a photo of a terrorist he saw in a newspaper. Since the patient was not in the military, didn't work for the government, and was politically uninvolved, there would be no reason for any foreign agent to be interested in him. Arguments were of no avail as the man had an unshakeable belief that, "Al Qaeda is after me."

A 75-year-old woman started a new drug for her PD. About one week later she became convinced that her husband was having an affair with the teenage girl who lived next door. When the husband argued that the couple was never apart so that the liason was physically impossible, the patient argued that, "You can't pull the wool over my eyes."

Delusions are usually the most bothersome side effect of drugs in PD, far more so than hallucinations. Luckily, they are much less common. Like the hallucinations, they are relatively stereotypic. Patients usually believe things that are bad or threatening. The single most common delusion is of spousal infidelity. Of course, this may in fact be occurring, but most of the time these are groundless complaints that are frequently impossible because the two are never out of sight of each other. Other common delusions are that strangers are living in the house, that people are entering the house and rearranging things, hiding objects, or stealing money. A particularly troublesome delusion is that impostors have been substituted for important family members and caregivers. Thus, the wife is not the "real" wife, but someone who looks, sounds, and acts like the real wife. The nurse is someone else, as are the children, and so on. Obviously one can't argue that this makes no sense, since the patient who believes this is not rational.

An 55-year-old Jewish woman who has had PD for 15 years, lives in a chronic care hospital and reports that the roof is used as a crematorium, and that body parts are being sold in other parts of the hospital. She believes that this is being done by Nazis and, as a result, takes to going to both Protestant and Catholic services each Sunday to fool them.

This unfortunate person lives in constant terror that she will be called next by an ongoing extension of the Holocaust of World War II. While obviously very contrived and based on absolutely no evidence, she nevertheless has a fixed delusional system, a set of beliefs that doesn't change.

A retired electrical engineering professor is convinced that people are secretly entering his house and performing some type of mischief. He knows this because he can hear them moving around or whispering. He refuses his doctor's attempts to lower his PD medication because he doesn't believe the doctor's reassurances that the sounds are hallucinations and his fixed belief is a delusion. During a hospitalization for a surgical problem unrelated to his PD, his PD medications are stopped. When the neurologist visits him, the doctor learns that the hallucinations have stopped. The patient no longer hears the voices. The doctor notes triumphantly that stopping the medication resulted in an end to the hallucinations. "Did anyone ever study the effect of this medication on hearing? I think that the PD medication makes me hear better. I think I can't hear those guys anymore because I'm a little deaf from not taking the medication."

This patient suffered from hallucinations, but he was also delusional, having fixed beliefs about his hallucinations. Even when the hallucinations resolved he maintained that they would be there if the medication allowed him to hear better. Whether hallucinating or not, he was still very smart.

Being psychotic doesn't mean being simple-minded. Smart people have the same thinking problems as average people, but they can come up with more sophisticated explanations for their behavior and thus cover up better.

Psychotic symptoms are more stressful for caregivers than motor problems. In fact, it has been recorded that caregiver stress is lower if the patient is wheelchair bound and unable to provide much self-help but is behaviorally intact, than if the patient is physically independent but has behavior problems. I think there can be little so devastating to a devoted spouse, having spent years in selfless effort to make life better for a loved one, than to then be accused of infidelity. That can be the last straw.

Some delusions are not paranoid and may even be pleasant: A trip to Florida the day before, an unexpected visit from some distant grandchildren, an interesting day at work, all while residing in a wheelchair at home or in the nursing home. These are not very stressful to those around them, but they still can be difficult, for example, if a caregiver is repetitively asked about the plans for tomorrow's trip which is never going to take place.

An 83-year-old man who lives at home asks his wife every day if she's bought the tickets for the trip to Florida. They had gone to Florida every winter for about a decade until the difficulties of the trip, and the man's recurrent problems waking up at night in a panic at not knowing where he was, made the trip counterproductive. No matter how many times the wife explains that they haven't gone to Florida for three winters and aren't going now either, this becomes a recurrent refrain, sometimes together with comments on the latest trip.

This type of delusion—that he is about to go on this trip and that he has recently been south—is not upsetting to the patient himself. This is unlike the vignettes I recounted above, in which the delusion upsets everyone. In this delusion the patient doesn't feel threatened and actually experiences some pleasure in the anticipation of the event. Oftentimes there may be a hint of anxiety as the patient obsesses a bit over the arrangements. Were the tickets purchased in time? Were they going to cost too much?

Delusions mostly develop in PD patients who are also suffering hallucinations, but not always.

DELUSIONS IN SCHIZOPHRENIA

The delusions in PD patients are not like those most commonly found in schizophrenia or other psychiatric disorders. In schizophrenia people may have delusions of grandeur, in which they think that they have special powers, that they are the next Napoleon or have been endowed with special powers from God. They frequently believe that other people can hear their thoughts, that others can steal their thoughts or even insert thoughts into their heads. Thus they may feel that they are thinking foreign thoughts that are not really their own. They often feel that people are spying on them, that their phones are bugged, or that cameras capture their every move so they must be devious in performing certain activities. Other unusual delusions include beliefs that parts of their bodies are diseased or malformed in some way, that they are rotting from within, that their arm isn't working the way it's supposed to, or that there are foreign objects in their body. Perhaps aliens from other planets have inserted special equipment to control their thoughts or movements. They may believe that characters on TV are delivering special coded messages to them via the TV or that strangers in crowds are similarly delivering messages via secret code to them, for example, that a sneeze may be a signal to begin a complex military operation. There is a website that sells special aluminum hats to counter the effects of alien radio signals meant to control people's brains.

While we all believe, especially when we're teenagers, that everyone is watching us, paying attention to our clothes and how we behave, we usually learn that most people don't care. A common paranoid delusion is that people are talking about you, or laughing at you behind your back.

PD patients do not experience these types of delusions, not unless they also have schizophrenia. How can you tell? Most often schizophrenia begins in early adulthood, in the late teens or early twenties, whereas PD usually begins in the sixth or seventh decade. It is possible to have both diseases, but the schizophrenia will always predate the onset of the PD. If a person develops what seems like both conditions at the same time, it is highly likely that the disease is not PD but rather some rare metabolic condition that may look like PD on a neurological exam.

EVALUATION

PD patients may hide their delusions very well, just as they hide their hallucinations. They may be very much aware that other people may find their delusions "crazy," so they don't talk about them. I will never forget the patient I asked to allow me to videotape a structured evaluation I was doing to illustrate how to perform the evaluation for a research study. I knew the patient had been suffering from hallucinations so I asked if I could record the evaluation in which I asked a large number of questions printed on a form.

She was, on the surface, a very well kept, intelligent, rational, normal-seeming person who had mild PD. She had told me about seeing cats that were a bit bothersome to her, and occasionally seeing some other animals, but I had no idea that she had delusions. When I asked if she ever felt things on her skin that weren't really there, she told me that she felt cockroaches and mice crawling on her when she went to sleep at night and how terrible this felt. I was amazed. Why hadn't I known this? But then it got worse. Did she feel other things? Well, yes, sometimes she felt the devil touch her. Then it turned out that the devil actually raped her, that her son was actually the devil's. And on and on. This patient had been under the care of a psychiatrist while concurrently under my own, but I had no idea of the depth of her mental illness. As Yogi Berra might have observed, "You can hear a lot just by listening." In this case it was actually not completely true. One learned a lot by *asking*. Without being asked, many patients will not volunteer sensitive information.

Delusions are similar to hallucinations in this regard. Patients often don't want others to think they're "crazy." In addition, since the delusions tend to be paranoid, patients may be even more reluctant to share these thoughts since the doctor may mock them, or side with the "others" who are spying, or simply ignore them, making the patient feel slighted. Patients who think their spouses are unfaithful are especially reluctant to tell this to the doctor, especially because they do not believe this is a medication side effect. Sometimes the patient thinks the doctor is part of the scheme to bring harm. One of my patients expressed the belief that my nurse was the devil and that his primary care doctor and I were part of a plan to harm him. Unfortunately he believed this about all his caretakers, so it became increasingly difficult to care for him.

DELUSIONS WITH PARTIAL INSIGHT

As patients begin to recover from an illness with delusions, they begin to develop insight into the illogicality of their delusion. A typical first step on the way to improvement would be a PD patient who says that he thinks his wife is cheating on him, but he knows this can't be true since he's with her all the time. Nevertheless, even though he knows from a rational perspective that this couldn't be happening, he nevertheless still feels as if she is seeing the next door neighbor. The patient has insight into the medication causing this effect and realizes that his belief will soon, hopefully, be replaced by the patient's premorbid mental state.

TREATMENT

Help, I'm currently battling three psychiatrists who insist on using haloperidol to treat psychosis in PD. One of these psychiatrists is the medical director for psychiatry here (***general Hospital). I've presented both with information about the manufacturer's contraindication for this usage and suggested the use of atypicals instead. My basic problem is that we've just decentralized to our mental health floors and I'm trying to establish a relationship with these docs. I would like to present them with information that reinforces this contraindication. From my reading, haloperidol is not an option in PD. The medical director of psychiatry believes the reason haloperidol is contraindicated is that it exacerbates parkinsonian symptoms, and that this is more appropriately a warning than an absolute contraindication. He believes that the only requirement for usage of haloperidol in PD is that dopamimetics must be adjusted to compensate for its negative effects. What I'd like to know is if any of you see haloperidol used for this indication and if you can share with me information or an approach I can use with these psychiatrists.

XXX, RPh, in an e-mail to his former Pharmacy instructor, 4/02.

Unlike the case with hallucinations, which are usually tolerated without problem, delusions almost always cause distress, in large part because they tend to be paranoid, and paranoia is an extremely unpleasant feeling, especially in someone who may not be fully independent.

The first approach to dealing with delusions, as with hallucinations, is to try to reduce the medications causing the problem. This means reducing or eliminating some of the medications taken for PD. At some point, these medications cannot be reduced without causing intolerable problems with mobility. At this point an antipsychotic medication must be introduced.

All of the drugs that treat psychotic symptoms block the effects, of dopamine to some degree. The first generation of antipsychotic drugs, that is, all the drugs used to treat schizophrenia until clozapine was released in 1992, caused parkinsonism as a side effect of blocking dopamine. Normal patients on these drugs looked like they had PD, and when the drugs were given to people who actually had PD their motor symptoms got worse, sometimes much worse.

As you can see from the e-mail I received a few years ago, this is still happening. I see this all too often. The newer generation of antipyschotic drugs, called "atypical antipsychotics," are less likely to cause parkinsonism or the other movement disorders that the first generation does, but unfortunately, they still do—with two exceptions. As of this writing, only quetiapine and clozapine are safe in terms of motor function. Some PD patients can take the other antipsychotic drugs without a problem, but many cannot. Unfortunately, after the motor function worsens, the patient may take weeks to recover after the drug is stopped. Virtually all American PD experts use only quetiapine or clozapine to treat this problem if the drugs causing the delusions can't be reduced or stopped.

If possible, it is best to not hospitalize the patient as changes of environment frequently exacerbate the problems, but this may be necessary if the patient is a threat to others or himself, or if his poor compliance makes it unlikely that he will improve at home or that the caretaker cannot cope with the demands.

Sometimes patients will refuse to go to the hospital and may be rational enough that they can't be forced against their will. In such cases it is best to withhold all PD medications. This "drug holiday" will help get the bad chemicals out of the brain, and will also make the patient less able to get into trouble, as his mobility worsens. As the psychiatric side effects wear off, the patient will usually see the advantage of being treated for the delusions. It may be important to also start either quetiapine (Seroquel) or clozapine (Clozaril) at very low doses.

Patients who recover from their psychotic symptoms will recall them. This is unlike the situation with delirium (confusion), which patients will remember as if it were a dream, with partial or little recall. They will recall very unpleasant experiences.

10

Confusion and Delirium

The word *delirium* has a technical meaning that describes a transient but significant worsening of mental function, with disorientation and a reduced, often fluctuating level of attention. *Confusion* is a nontechnical term that sometimes means the same thing, but also refers to a long-term but relatively stable condition with decreased memory and thinking. Parkinson's disease (PD) patients become delirious either because of their medications or because of medical illnesses, usually infections. A sudden mental change almost always is the result of one of these two processes.

The term *confusion* is a general term. Families will use it to describe a sudden change, a chronic state with fluctuations, or a chronic stable condition. They usually mean that the person is disoriented and behaves in a manner that is different from what used to be his normal behavior. Some families get used to a stable level of disorientation, especially in someone elderly, and consider it normal. This family will employ the term confusion to refer to episodes where the patient is far more confused than is usual.

*A*n 80-year-old woman lives with her son and his family. She *never goes out by herself. She prepares her own meals to a limited degree but keeps to a schedule of her own that doesn't vary from day to day, including taking her own medications. Sometimes, though, in the evening she wonders aloud where she is, and when she can go home.*

This patient appears to suffer from "sundowning," getting confused at night, when the sun goes down. This is currently a stable problem for her, but will slowly worsen.

*A*74-year-old man recently retired and was thought to have no *problems with his memory or thinking, but on a vacation trip in which he stayed at a hotel, he awoke in the middle of the night and couldn't find the bathroom. He woke his wife asking who had moved the bathroom.*

This man may simply have panicked, awakening at night, not recalling where he was. It could also be the first sign of dementia, a permanent and increasing loss of memory.

We think of confusional states as occurring intermittently or chronically. What does this mean? Chronic confusion is equivalent to being demented. These people are disoriented to some degree all the time and cannot remember well. Some people who seem completely normal most of the time suddenly act in a confused or odd manner, which may be due to new medications, intoxication from alcohol or other substances (older people do drink alcohol to excess or use drugs, just as younger people do), while others with a stable degree of confusion sometimes become even more confused.

DELIRIUM

The technical definition of delirium requires an alteration in the level of consciousness, so that the person is usually less alert than

• • • • • • • • • • • • •   DELIRIUM   • • • • • • • • • • • • • •

Reduced clarity or awareness of the environment

Reduced ability to focus attention

Reduced ability to sustain attention

Reduced ability to understand events at the person's usual level

Reduced ability to solve problems or respond with the baseline
    level of intellectual skills

The condition evolves over hours to days.

The condition fluctuates during each day.

The delirium is the result of a medical disorder or drug
    intoxication.

• •

normal, but possibly hypervigilant, with a reduced clarity of awareness
of the environment, and reduced ability to focus, sustain, or shift attention. There is also a change in the ability to understand or solve problems. The condition evolves over hours to days, fluctuates during each
day, and results from some identifiable medical disorder.

CONFUSION IN A DEMENTED PERSON

People who have any degree of cognitive or memory problems are
at higher risk for confusional spells. Oftentimes the baseline abnormality
in thinking only becomes recognized after the first episode of confusion.

*A 76-year-old woman is described as being "sharp as a tack."
The night before, however, she had become agitated about an
intruder in the house, called the police, and acted irrationally when
they arrived, accusing them of "being in cahoots" with the thief.
The patient is admitted to the hospital and found to have normal
blood work, a normal brain CT scan, but has mild problems with
orientation, giving the wrong month, year, and season, and is not
able to recall her hospital room number despite being told several
times.*

This patient has mild dementia that was not recognized by the family. By keeping to a fairly unchanging routine, she was able to perform all her activities of daily life without fail. It is likely that her family did not engage her in discussions requiring sophisticated knowledge, current events, or abstract thinking that would have revealed her problems earlier.

Just like little children, the elderly, particularly those with some degree of dementia, are subject to confusional spells with infections and especially with fevers, even when the infection is unrelated to the brain. Even minor infections may cause an elderly person with dementia to suddenly become much worse. Sometimes this is seen in the form of lethargy and increased sleepiness, but also with confusional spells that can be very scary to the rest of the family. Often, when this happens the first time, the patient is brought to the emergency department where the family is told that the patient has probably had a "mini-stroke." This is almost never the case, since strokes hardly ever cause confusional states. In most cases the confusion is due either to an "occult" (hidden, or unrecognized) infection, or to medication, possibly taken incorrectly. One should never forget that alcohol and pain medications may be the cause, even when the patient was thought to have stopped taking alcohol years before. Rarely, some other medical problem is recognized. Usually in these cases it is either a kidney or liver problem, some of which may then secondarily cause difficulty metabolizing medications, rendering them toxic even though the dosing hasn't changed.

CONFUSION

It is important to recognize that a variety of "natural" uncontrollable things may cause confusion. Firstly, people with dementia often fluctuate on their own, regardless of what's going on in their surroundings. In people with PD, the medication levels in the blood rise and fall, often in ways that differ daily even though the same medications are taken at the same time, simply because gut motility, that is,

· · · · · · · · · · CAUSES OF "CONFUSION" · · · · · · · · · ·

Infection

Fever

Medication error

New medication

Withdrawal from medication

Overuse of pain medication

Change of environment

     Sleeping in a new setting

     Change in caretaker

Falls, even if sparing the head

Kidney or liver problems

Declines in oxygen due to lung problems

Periods of low blood pressure

Alcohol

Vivid dream/nightmare

REM intrusion

Hallucinations

Anxiety

Seizure or postseizure state

Hypoglycemia

Thyroid disease

· ·

the speed of intestinal movements may vary over the course of a day as well as from day to day.

People with dementia will have a degree of confusion that varies with their level of sleepiness. After a good night's sleep the patient may function better than normal, but might feel run down by the afternoon, and improve again after a brief nap. Anxiety frequently worsens mental confusion, as do environmental changes (for example, sleeping away from home or rearranging furniture).

Patients with the disorder dementia with Lewy bodies (DLB; see Chapter 7) often have fluctuations in their mental processes during each day. This may also happen in PD patients who become demented. The presence of the fluctuations is one of the defining traits of DLB. It is unknown why these fluctuations occur, but patients not only become more or less confused, but they may also have periods in which they become unresponsive, as if in a coma but with the eyes open. These spells may last over 30 minutes and are extremely unnerving.

CONFUSIONAL SPELLS IN PATIENTS WITHOUT AN UNDERLYING DEMENTIA

PD patients who have an episode of confusion have a similar list of possible explanations for their spell as the demented patient, but the likelihood of finding an explanation is much higher if the person is not demented. In addition, the environmental explanations, such as a change in caregiver or a change in the physical environment, are much less likely to cause this in a nondemented patient, and an "organic" or medical explanation is far more likely to be found as a cause.

Infection is the first possible cause to consider. Most people with infections have symptoms, but not always. An infection in the lungs usually causes cough and sputum production, along with a fever, but not always. Sometimes there is chest pain or shortness of breath, but occasionally lung infections will cause no obvious symptoms and shows up only as confusional states. Bladder and kidney infections are very common and may cause confusion as well. Women are generally far more likely to develop bladder infections than men, but as men age and develop prostate enlargement, they are at risk for bladder as well as prostate infections, both of which may contribute to confusional spells. Other organs are rarely infected, so the basic medical evaluation requires a chest x-ray, or chest exam by a doctor, and a urinalysis.

Other medical conditions may contribute. During the warm summer months dehydration causes some frail patients to become confused. Kidney failure, even if mild, can alter the excretion of amantadine, a commonly used medication in PD, so that even before anyone becomes aware that the kidney isn't functioning properly the

patient begins to hallucinate and act confused. It is because the amantadine has built up to toxic levels and has intoxicated or poisoned the
patient. The amantadine is not harming the kidney and did not cause
the kidney problem.

A *60-year-old patient taking L-Dopa and amantadine starts
to see little children in his bedroom at night. The next day
he asks his wife where his wife is. He also wants to know when
his son is visiting, although his son lives in another state and just
made plans with the patient to visit next month. She brings the
patient to the primary care provider who finds that the creatinine,
one measure of kidney function, is double what it had been a few
months earlier, and determines that the patient has mild kidney
failure. Over the next three days the kidney problem fails to improve
but the amantadine was stopped on admission to the hospital, and
on the third day mental function returned to normal even though
the kidneys were not yet working at full strength. They had been
working well enough to clear the amantadine from the body.*

The medications used in PD are not broken down by the liver so
that liver problems do not usually cause particular problems in
PD, but moderate degrees of liver dysfunction will cause confusion
in any person, with PD or not.

The first thing to do in assessing a confusional spell is to obtain
a complete history. Did it occur at night or during the day? Where
did the spell occur? If it occurred away from home, like a relative's
house or a hotel, then the chances are that it was due to the environmental change. Did it occur at night? Perhaps it was a very realistic dream or nightmare since many people with PD, especially those
taking L-Dopa, often experience dreams that seem particularly real.
When they awaken from the dream they may believe the dream really
occurred. Some PD patients act out certain dreams, particularly
dreams of fighting or running away. During the dream the patient may

hit, flail, kick, yell, or even sleepwalk. These spells may also look like confusional states (see REM sleep behavior disorder in Chapter 12).

A 63-year-old man with PD, taking L-Dopa, ropinerole, and selegiline, awakens at night to investigate some noises that he thinks he heard, certain that the neighbors' house is burning down. He wants to call 911, but his wife insists that they look out the window first, to prove that there is no fire.

In this case the man apparently had a vivid dream, so real that he acted on it and wanted to call the fire department. Many people would call this "confusion" and bring such a person to the emergency department of their local hospital.

Not all confusional spells require an evaluation, although the first episode does. If the spells establish a pattern, then further evaluations after the first one are not usually worthwhile. However, the first thing to do is to decide if the spell is indeed an episode of "confusion." A single spell, lasting only a few minutes, is quite different from several hours of sustained abnormal behavior.

EVALUATION OF CONFUSIONAL SPELLS

After the history is obtained to determine if the spell was a sleep-related problem, or an environmentally triggered event, or if symptoms of an infection may be present, a chest x-ray, urinalysis, blood count (looking for signs of an infection), and tests of kidney and liver function and electrolytes are obtained. These are far more important than imaging studies such as a computerized tomography (CT) scan or magnetic resonance imaging (MRI), as the problems that cause confusion are virtually always due to "toxic/metabolic" problems, meaning that they are due to some type of poisoning of the brain, not to tumors, blood clots, or strokes.

On rare occasions an electroencephalogram (EEG, or "brain wave" test) may be useful. Seizures are usually quite obvious. Most patients with seizures will stiffen and shake, and will either become unconscious or display an impaired level of consciousness; however, some will have only changes in their behavior. Although seizures usually last between thirty seconds and one minute, and only occasionally longer, there are uncommon seizures that last for extended periods of time and cause a "twilight" mental state. Such patients are not usually interactive and therefore will not usually engage in conversations. They will look as if they are in another world, as if they are communicating with you through a barrier of some sort.

However, it is common for people to have confusional states *after* a seizure. These are called "postictal" states, since the term "ictal" means an attack or sudden spell, which a seizure is. The postictal state usually lasts far longer than the seizure, so that a seizure of one minute may be followed by a 30-minute postictal confusional state. Rarely, the confusion may last for hours or even days following a seizure. It is therefore possible for a person to occasionally have an unwitnessed or unnoticed seizure followed by a lengthy confusional postictal state. In most cases a patient will not be aware that she has had a seizure, unless there are tell-tale happenings that the patient has learned to identify as the hallmark of a recent seizure, things such as urinary incontinence, tongue maceration from chewing on the tongue during the seizure, headache, confusion, or bilateral shoulder or sometimes leg or back pain from the extreme exertion during a seizure.

It is sometimes a good idea to check for extraneous drugs, a so-called tox screen, meaning a "toxicology" (poison) screen. In some cases patients will hide their alcohol intake, insisting that they don't drink or drink only very small amounts on social occasions, but will then turn out to be fairly significant alcoholics. The patient may consider their alcohol intake small, compared to usage decades ago, but with age plus several medications that older patients and PD patients in particular take, the tolerance is markedly reduced. Narcotics also show up on toxicology screens so that the person who takes too much of their pain pills, or accidentally takes a few of their spouse's pain pills, may end up confused. Unfortunately, it is not possible to obtain blood levels of the medications used for treating PD. If one could, then we'd be able to tell if a patient accidentally took too much of their medications, inadvertently overdosing.

A very important fact that most doctors don't appreciate is that delirium in an older patient may take several weeks to resolve, not simply hours or days, which should be borne in mind when the previously mentally intact older PD patient becomes delirious but does not return to normal in the first few days after treatment. The patient will sometimes be labeled as having dementia because he doesn't improve, but really may still be delirious.

Compulsive Behavior

Although there was a report in 1995 describing a seemingly rare problem caused by medications, it wasn't until around 2005 that the Parkinson's disease (PD) community began to appreciate that the dopamine agonist drugs occasionally caused problems with compulsive behaviors, particularly gambling, shopping, sex, and eating.

When I started writing the first edition of this book I did not have this chapter in my plans. I was aware of compulsive behaviors being a side effect of the treatment for PD, but I thought it was very rare, and although worth mentioning in passing, not worth spending too much attention on. That was until one of the articles on compulsive gambling made the news and patients starting coming out of the woodwork, reporting that they had never told me about this problem because they were either embarrassed or did not think that it was related to either their PD or to their medications. After they saw it described in the newspaper, they realized the connection and brought it to my attention.

A compulsion is an activity performed to relieve a severe feeling of anxiety. Therefore, compulsions are classified as anxiety disorders. By performing the activity, psychic stress is relieved. If the activity is not performed the patient becomes increasingly anxious. A certain degree of compulsive behavior is helpful. You want your surgeon, for example, to be compulsive, to make sure that every suture is tied perfectly, that all the gauze pads are accounted for, that all the tissues that should be sewn together are. You certainly want your airplane mechanic to be very compulsive. On the other hand, if the mechanic is unwilling to allow a plane to be cleared unless he checks everything 50 times, the plane will never be approved for fight. You want your children to be clean and neat, but you don't want them to be incapacitated because every item has to be at right angles to every other item, and you don't want any piece of lint on the floor to be a cause for extreme agitation.

Probably the most well-known compulsion in the popular mind is hand washing. We see that on TV or in the movies. In the movie, *The Aviator*, Howard Hughes suffered from a severe compulsive disorder and was incapacitated by the need for cleanliness. Compulsive behavior relieves tension, even though it may also create it. For example, the person who must return to his house to make sure he closed all the windows, despite having checked the windows 15 times, knows he will be late for an appointment, but simply can't leave. He must then check that he locked the door, and once away from the house, return to be certain that it really was locked.

Compulsive gambling as a side effect of medication is a new observation. It certainly took me by surprise, despite the fact that I was the first person to report a very bizarre behavior in some of my PD patients, called "punding," which is a primitive compulsive behavior disorder. "Punding" was first reported in patients who were addicted to amphetamines ("uppers" or stimulants) or cocaine. The addicts, when high, would spend their time taking apart and putting back together (although they were not so good with the putting back together part!) objects such as flashlights, radios, and other objects that had several parts. They will do this over and over again for hours and reportedly do not like being disturbed during this ritualistic behavior. They find it relaxing and fulfilling.

In PD we described patients who repetitively catalogued collections of jewelry, even though there weren't many pieces in the collection; a patient who tallied sums of numbers over and over again and couldn't stop although he could easily produce the answer to the sum he had added hundreds of times; a patient who was unable to stop reading labels on cans when she went into the supermarket and therefore not only couldn't shop, but couldn't accompany her family when they went shopping.

A 50-year-old woman with an eight-year history of PD reported that after a recent increase in her ropinerole she began to shop "compulsively." Actually, her problem was the opposite. She became unable to purchase anything. The problem she developed was that she felt compelled to always get the absolute best price on whatever she bought. When she tried to buy something she would end up having to check the price at several different stores scattered all over the state. By the end of the day she knew the prices everywhere, but still couldn't buy anything. She thus became an inefficient shopper who could not make up her mind, and perhaps the opposite of a compulsive shopper—a compulsive comparison shopper.

A 35-year-old man with PD began gambling, a problem he had overcome before the onset of PD. In addition, however, while lying to me about his gambling, he began to collect lawnmower motors, and then to start using crack cocaine. He traded his car for crack. After being arrested by the police, he confessed everything to me, triggering a major change in his medication and a referral to a psychiatrist with a strong background in PD.

When a problem like this is described, the first question to ask is whether it is part of PD, due to the medications or whether it is even related to PD at all. After all, most people at the gambling casinos do not have PD, do not take a dopamine agonist, and are not gambling compulsively. In the case of PD, however, we find that patients who never gambled started to gamble after their medication doses were raised and stopped gambling when the doses were lowered. Interestingly, unlike the situation with most drug-induced behavioral changes, the urge to gamble was not viewed as an alien, or foreign, feeling. The patients, out of the blue, suddenly become interested in gambling, just like they might suddenly become interested in Civil War history, architecture, reading mystery stories, or knitting.

A PD patient who had been a part-time artist stopped working due to PD disability and began to paint full time. Whereas before she had painted a few hours each week, she was now painting several hours each day. Her painting style did not change, but she now felt a "calling" to art. Art became her passion, and she felt that being an artist was what she had been born to do. However, she did not stop caring for herself. She maintained her usual social activities, her household chores, managed her finances acceptably, and did not withdraw from the world to pursue her art to the exclusion of everything else. Her doctors thought this marked increase in her devotion to art represented a medication effect.

This is a very interesting case, because it illustrates the difficulty of determining if a certain behavior is pathological or not, and, if it is pathological, whether it is disease related or something we might see in the general population. I view this vignette as illustrating the rare circumstance of PD being a "liberating" force. A person who had been constrained by a full-time job now has the time to pursue a lifelong ambition. I do not regard her increased interest in art as pathological.

If the artist had suddenly stopped caring for herself, found it impossible to leave the canvas in order to go to the toilet, or to eat, or to see friends and family, I would deem it pathological. In this case I am reminded of one of my patients who had a severe tremor. He had to give up his business as a glazier. After all, how can you cut and mount glass with a bad tremor? When I commiserated with him over his having to sell a business he had developed over a few decades he told me that this was a great opportunity. What he really liked to do was umpire amateur baseball games and this gave him a lot more time for that. And he spent the next several spring and summers doing exactly that. He was not on a dopamine agonist. He was following his "calling." This artist had a calling. She was not the victim of a compulsive disorder.

When we find that a "new" behavior disorder is more common than we expect, we need to find out if it really is more common. Sometimes we are confused by random chance. I once saw five cases of spinal cord stroke within one year in a small community hospital. This was a staggeringly high number of cases and I reported them. Since it was a small hospital we had good records on all the other stroke cases so we assumed that five must be the usual number for a year. As it turns out, those five were the only ones I've seen in over thirty years. They just happened to cluster, causing me to misunderstand the epidemiology of the condition. So when we find some PD patients developing a gambling habit, we must determine if this is similar to the general population. Maybe the same number of people of similar age also gamble, and maybe they too develop it in their later years?

Several studies have now clearly shown that these "impulse control disorders" (ICD) are quite clearly linked to the dopamine agonists (bromocriptine, pramipexole, ropinerole, and rotigotine). In PD patients, and ICD occurs in about 10% to 15% of patients, and many patients may experience more than one, for example gambling and hypersexuality.

OTHER COMPULSIVE ACTIVITIES

Any activity can be "overdone" and incorporated into a compulsive ritual. So far in PD they have been primarily limited to gambling, shopping, eating, sexual preoccupation, and punding, but a large number of other, often unusual compulsions have been described. "Consumerism" (compulsive shopping or spending excess money) tends to occur in women, just as hypersexuality tends to occur in men, but both occur in both genders.

A patient who was an avid fisherman, who travelled around the country visiting friends in order to fish with them, began injuring himself by fishing off rocks on the beach, even during the winter in Rhode Island. He fished every day, often in inclement conditions.

This patient had always fished a lot and his fishing seemed excessive to me, but this wasn't my hobby, and I could only counsel him to keep safe. We stopped his ropinerole because of dyskinesias, and when he returned, he told me that his fishing had been a compulsive problem, that he still fished, but just as he had done before. He no longer felt the need to fish every day, whether unsafe or inclement.

A patient ice fishes for three days straight in New Hampshire (and does not drink alcohol).

Another patient bakes a cherry pie every evening, which he does not eat, because he doesn't like cherry pies.

A 60-year-old man speeds when he drives his car so that his wife refuses to be a passenger with him at the wheel.

An elderly man spends most of his day polishing pennies.

An older woman cleans her oven all day, every day.

In each case, unless the behavior resolves with a reduction in the drug treatment, it will be unclear if the behavior is induced by the medications or simply developed in the PD patient in an unrelated manner. Lightning may indeed strike twice.

Because these activities may seem normal to the patient, and even to the family, and because they are perceived more as character flaws than as medication or disease side effects, they are not brought to the doctor's attention. They should be, and a polite inquiry as to whether this may be a medication side effect should be made.

Treatment varies. Obviously the first approach should be to lower the dopamine agonist, but this may cause worsened parkinsonism, and the patient may prefer to gamble or have the compulsion than to be stiff and immobile. Trials of other dopamine agonists, or substitutes may be tried. Nondopaminergic substitutes are likely to be successful at eliminating the behavior, but may not make up for the lost benefit in mobility. Drugs for obsessive-compulsive disorder, such as sertraline (Zoloft), fluoxetine (Prozac), and paroxetine (Paxil) work for some patients, but not for most, just as quetiapine (Seroquel), a drug for schizophrenia may also be tried, but is usually not very helpful. In some cases, deep brain stimulation surgery was used to reduce the need for PD medication. Once the dopamine agonists was stopped, the behavior resolved.

The first step in treatment is recognizing the extent of the problem and the connection with the PD medication. Unless the patient or the family is informed, they won't link this behavior change to the medication and will not inform the doctor. The doctor needs to ask about the behavior, and not all doctors are aware of the issue. Furthermore, one aspect of the problem is that the patients often underestimate the extent of the problem and often behave like drug addicts and alcoholics, who deny they have a problem and tend to minimize their behavior. I have seen patients lose their entire retirement income as a result of this problem being unrecognized. It is important for a family member to accompany the patient to the doctor visit to accurately describe the problem because the patient will often deny that there is a problem or will say that it's now "under control." Occasional marriages and stable relationships will dissolve when the PD patient becomes hypersexual and either makes uncomfortable demands or goes outside the relationship for sexual release.

DOPAMINE DYSREGULATION SYNDROME

This is a much less common problem than ICD, but probably much harder to treat. In the dopamine dysregulation syndrome (DDS), the patient behaves like an addict, using excessive amounts of L-Dopa. This disorder occurs primarily with L-Dopa. Patients will report that they need more drug because they are increasingly bothered by "off" period immobility and discomfort, but no matter how many times each day they take their L-Dopa, they always want more. The problem comes to a head when the large doses start causing behavior problems. Usually the behavior is psychotic, with hallucinations and paranoid delusions, but sometimes the problem is anxiety. In fact, the patient appears to be taking the L-Dopa in response to anxiety, but it is not clear that the L-Dopa makes the anxiety better. Drug addicts feel better when they take their drug, whether heroin, cocaine, amphetamine, or something else. The PD patients do not get high. One of my patients would hoard his pills and then binge. When he lived at home he got arrested more than once because the excess L-Dopa would make him hallucinate that his neighbors were having a party, so he would knock on their door at 2 a.m. and ask to come in.

This is a very difficult problem to solve. Patients need to take L-Dopa. It is our best medication for treating PD, and when patients say they "need" the drug, I believe that they are truly hurting. It is very hard to tell a PD patient who is "off" that he cannot take the pill that will relieve his discomfort. The problem is that it doesn't work for very long and the drug-seeking behavior continues. Generally, this is dealt with by combined use of L-Dopa and other PD medications, and having someone other than the patient control the medications.

12

. . . .

Sleep

Parkinson's disease (PD) patients have a variety of sleep problems, which include excessive daytime sleepiness (EDS), poor sleeping at night, difficulty falling asleep, difficulty staying asleep, abnormal sleep behaviors, abnormal dreaming, dreaming while awake, obstructive sleep apnea, and overactive bladder.

NORMAL SLEEP

Normal people sleep about six to nine hours every day, usually at night. The range of what is necessary to maintain normal alertness varies considerably from one person to another. The time when people want to go to sleep or when they awaken in the morning also varies considerably. For most people, the amount of time slept in a 24-hour period is fairly fixed, so that if someone naps during the day, that person will probably sleep less at night.

Most people take about 20 to 40 minutes to fall asleep, but there is a large variation across the population and a large variation in any particular person from day to day. If you sleep poorly one night you'll probably sleep better the next. If you work or exercise very hard you'll probably sleep better than usual. If you're worried about something or you drink more alcohol than usual, you'll probably not sleep very soundly. People move about in bed and change their position about every 15 to 30 minutes.

There are four stages of sleep: Two of light sleep, one of heavy sleep, and dream sleep. There is a structure to these stages of sleep so that "normal" sleep consists of a certain amount of time in one stage, followed by time in another, then another, and so on. During normal sleep, people cycle through these stages. Although most people do not remember their dreams, we all dream a few times each night in dream sleep that usually lasts less than 30 minutes at a time. Even the person who "never dreams" really just never remembers the dreams. The average person older than 50 years old dreams about four times each night, which is less than one-fourth of the night's sleep. Dream sleep usually doesn't begin until the patient has been asleep for about 90 minutes so that most naps are not associated with dreams.

Many drugs affect sleep. The most commonly used drug that affects sleep is alcohol but PD medications often cause daytime sleepiness, hence a tendency to nap and possibly less sleep at night.

EXCESSIVE DAYTIME SLEEPINESS

A very common problem in PD is excessive daytime sleepiness (EDS). This is also very common in the general population and is often measured by the Epworth Sleepiness Scale, which is a useful guide to determining whether someone sleeps enough at night or not. In fact, many Americans do not sleep sufficiently at night and, as a result, are sleepy during the day, sometimes causing driving accidents or poor performance at work or school.

In PD there are many reasons for sleepiness during the day. The medications, particularly the dopamine agonists (pramipexole, ropinerole, rotigotine, and bromocriptine), all may cause EDS. A very large percentage of PD patients have difficulty falling asleep, staying asleep, or getting good-quality, restful sleep.

On the mild end of the spectrum, patients will describe feeling fine while engaged, but fall asleep within minutes of sitting down to watch TV, or when reading a book. They can drive without a problem but tend to fall asleep if they're the passenger. At the other end of the spectrum some PD patients can't stay awake more than a few minutes at a time. Their spouses report that they fall asleep while eating or in the middle of a sentence.

Many PD patients are physically unable to pursue their old activities. They can't get into the car and drive to see friends and relatives. They can't go to the golf course, to the mall, to the movie theater, or work in the yard. They are pretty much stuck in the house reading and watching TV. This is boring, and boredom produces sleepiness, so they nap during the day, whether they want to or not.

An 80-year-old woman with PD complains that she's always falling asleep. Her walking is poor due to the PD and her severe arthritis. Although she loves to read, she reports that within 15 minutes of reading any book or magazine, she finds herself asleep. She falls asleep in front of the TV at 8 p.m., but then can't fall asleep when she goes to bed at 11 p.m. She gets out of bed at 8 a.m., feeling sleepy, and naps after breakfast.

I believe that EDS is greatly underappreciated in PD patients. I think it is a major contributing factor to the very common symptom of fatigue, but also contributes to impaired memory and thinking. We all know that we think our best after a good night's sleep. We advise our children to get a "good night's sleep" before their exams in school. In fact, medical training programs for doctors have taken this into account by restricting the number of hours a doctor can work in a 48-hour period. After a 24-hour stretch without sleep our thinking is about as impaired as if we had consumed two glasses of beer. How many people would want their surgeon to operate on them after a couple of beers? Similarly, after a poor night's sleep, or, more likely, several poor nights' sleep, the ability to concentrate, which is a primary requirement for

• • • • • •   REASONS FOR DAYTIME SLEEPINESS   • • • • • •

Sleepiness due to PD medications (pramipexole, ropinerole,
rotigotine, and bromocriptine)

Sleepiness due to L-Dopa, antianxiety medications, antidepressants,
antipsychotics, nighttime sleep medications

Poor nighttime sleeping
Difficulty falling asleep
Difficulty staying asleep
Poor quality sleep
Fragmented sleep

Abnormal sleep cycles
Boredom
Depression
Anxiety

• •

remembering new information, is seriously impaired. Our ability to solve problems, and, equally important, to avoid problems, is reduced with decreased sleep. Sometimes patients with memory problems actually have EDS.

EDS also contributes to depression and, most likely, to the development of psychosis and hallucinations.

A 76-year-old man seems fine during the day, but each night he gets up and wanders around the house looking for evidence that his house was burglarized. In the morning he gets out of bed feeling sleepy and never has the energy to do anything, preferring to stay home and nap while watching TV.

FALLING ASLEEP

PD patients may have trouble falling asleep for a number of reasons. The most common reason is difficulty becoming comfortable. Many PD patients have back or neck pain, either from arthritis or directly from their stooped postures. When they lie in bed they have problems searching for a comfortable position since turning in bed and moving around is so difficult. Turning over in bed with PD is like a turtle righting itself after being placed on its back. Some patients are bothered by their tremor, so they try to put the shaking body part, usually the fingers or hands, under something, like a hip, to keep it from moving. Chattering teeth from jaw tremor may be bothersome not only because of the movement itself, but also from the noise if the upper and lower teeth meet.

Patients who have been on L-Dopa for a few years frequently develop abnormal movements from the medication, and these can interfere with sleep too. Some of these movements are "dyskinesias," which are usually random fidgety movements, but more bothersome are "dystonic" postures, in which the toes curl or the feet turn. These can be painful and are, at best, uncomfortable. Some patients will experience "wearing off" from their medications, so that they get into bed while their medicine is working, but as they are trying to fall asleep, the medicine starts to wear off, making a formerly comfortable position newly uncomfortable.

Patients with severe neck stiffness may need many pillows to maintain their head in a comfortable position. And many PD patients, like people everywhere, have many things on their mind that make them worry. Anxiety interferes with falling asleep, as everyone knows.

Many medications alter sleep, some by increasing sleepiness during the day so that daytime naps make it difficult to fall asleep at a reasonable time at night, some by inducing stimulation. Probably the most commonly used drugs that interfere with sleep are the selective serotonin reuptake inhibitor (SSRI) antidepressant drugs and alcohol. I believe that the incidence of alcohol abuse by PD patients is extremely low, but it isn't zero and some patients do abuse this drug. Some PD patients take medications specifically to combat EDS. These drugs, of course, interfere with sleep. If a patient is overly sensitive, or if the dose is too high, or if the dose is taken later in the morning than ideal, the person may still have the antisleep effects when it's time to go to sleep for the night.

RESTLESS LEGS SYNDROME

This very common syndrome was first described in 1945, but didn't make its way to medical or public consciousness until the 1990s. Generally, patients with restless legs syndrome (RLS) describe an uncomfortable sensation in the legs that worsens at night, particularly when the person is resting, and is relieved by standing, walking, or rubbing the legs. The urge to move the legs is the single most common aspect of the syndrome. This is considered one of the most common neurological syndromes in the Western world.

RLS is often difficult to distinguish from akathisia, a syndrome discussed below. RLS frequently runs in families, frequently is associated with periodic leg movements (PLMs) of sleep (kicking movements during sleep), affects falling asleep and staying asleep, and generally responds nicely to the same medications as are used in treating PD itself. Interestingly, RLS seems to be more common in PD patients than in age-matched control populations. In many cases the RLS predates the onset of the PD; however, it is unclear how many of the RLS cases may actually have had akathisia. Some authorities believe that RLS and akathisia are, in fact, the same entity, but most authorities disagree. Certainly, however there is some overlap. RLS may be associated with low iron levels in the blood, so that certain laboratory studies may be necessary, particularly in a person who has a low red blood cell count (anemia). It is also associated with disorders of the peripheral nerves called "peripheral neuropathies," or simply, "neuropathies." An overactive thyroid can produce a restlessness that may be similar to RLS, although usually the restlessness doesn't just occur in the evenings.

Some patients with RLS also describe discomfort in other body parts than the legs, but in almost all cases the legs are also involved. About 80% of patients with RLS also have kicking movements during sleep.

• • • • • • • • • • RESTLESS LEGS SYNDROME • • • • • • • • • •

I. Required features
   The urge to move the legs due to unpleasant leg
      sensations such as crawling, tingling, aching
   Worsened symptoms when resting, either sitting
      or lying down
   Relief of leg discomfort with walking and moving
   Worsened symptoms at night or symptoms only at night

II. Helpful diagnostic features
   Family history of RLS
   Improvement with PD medications
   Periodic limb movements

III. Other features
   Normal examination
   Sleep problems
   Variable clinical course

• •

AKATHISIA

Akathisia is a term that was coined in 1902 by a psychiatrist who described two young women who he thought suffered from hysteria. They were unable to remain seated. The term means "unable to sit." He walked the grounds of the sanitarium with his charges, obtaining their histories and treating them. He considered this incessant walking a sign of their illness and found it so unusual that he felt compelled to describe it in the medical literature.

Interestingly, the problem had been recognized before but had not been given a name. The first reference I have found to this problem is in a textbook from the early 1900s which notes a comment in a yet earlier text from the 1800s describing a peculiar behavior in a chamberlain in the court of Napoleon III. This gentleman, who suffered from PD, violated court protocol by constantly sitting and standing to relieve his inner discomfort. It is not an easy syndrome to define so it is not clear how common it is in PD, but it appears to be quite common. In one study from Canada it was found to affect about 25% of PD patients.

Akathisia may occur in PD patients, both in the untreated as well as in the treated state. It may in fact be related to PD medication, most commonly as an "off" problem, that is, when the PD medications aren't working well. There are various definitions of the syndrome, but most agree that akathisia is a syndrome of inner restlessness, relieved by moving or walking.

STAYING ASLEEP

In my experience more PD people have problems staying asleep than falling asleep. They awaken for a number of reasons. Until quite recently it was standard teaching that tremors and other movements disappear during sleep. Even though patients would frequently tell me that their tremors woke them up, I told them that really they awoke for other reasons and that upon awakening their tremor restarted. Studies in the sleep lab proved that patients may start to shake when they are in the light stages of sleep. Tremors do not occur during the deeper levels of sleep or during dream sleep. In the lighter levels of sleep, however, the tremors may develop sufficiently to wake the person up.

Patients awaken because of the need to void. PD affects the bladder by making people feel the need to urinate more frequently than they used to. The bladder feels full when it is only partly full. In addition, PD patients often must urinate very quickly or they will have an accident. In fact, the bladder may start to contract, causing severe urgency and sometimes incontinence. Many PD patients have fluid accumulation in their legs. When they lie flat in bed the water that is in the legs starts to go back into the circulation, causing the kidneys to filter out this extra fluid, filling the bladder. Thus the legs act like sponges, soaking up water during the day, and at night, when the patient lies flat, the water drains from the "sponge" into the

• • • • • • MOVEMENT DISORDERS OCCURRING • • • • • •
DURING THE NIGHT

Tremor
Akinesia/bradykinesia
Rigidity
Painful dystonia
Dyskinesias
Akathisia
Periodic limb movements
Myoclonic jerks
Restless legs syndrome
REM sleep behavior disorder (RBD)

• •

(From Grandas F, Iranzo A. Nocturnal problems occurring in PD. *Neurology* 2004;63(Suppl 3):S8–S11).

bloodstream and then into the bladder. It's like drinking a gallon or two of water just before bedtime. What comes in must go out.

Everyone wakes up during sleep. Generally people just fall back to sleep. Usually someone wakes up or moves from a deep to a lighter level of sleep, moves around in bed a bit to get comfortable and goes back to a deeper level of sleep. Some people wake up several times during the night, but don't even know it because it is for a very brief time. Patients with sleep apnea, for example, may awaken hundreds of time each night, but not recall a single episode. For the PD patient who awakens, however, turning over and moving are difficult. What might be a two-second arousal for a normal person may be a hellish hour for the person with PD.

One of the unusual reasons for PD patients to awaken is sleep talking. Many PD patients yell, laugh, talk, cry, or even sing in their sleep. Sometimes the talker awakens himself with the noise, but far more common, the talker remains asleep but the bed partner awakens.

Once awake most people then feel the urge to void, which creates a new series of problems because by the time this occurs, the effects of the PD medications have generally worn off. This means that getting out of bed is a big production, followed by shuffling to the toilet, shuffling back to bed, and trying to get comfortable again.

Many PD patients end up sleeping in an easy chair in front of the TV.

PERIODIC LEG MOVEMENTS

PLMs are very common in the general population, especially among the elderly. The movements may occur while awake, as well as during sleep. These are slow kicking movements. They usually bother the bed partner more than the patient but they may awaken the patient as well. These movements are often associated with RLS and respond to the same medications.

DREAM SLEEP PROBLEMS

There are two problems that PD patients have that few other people have. One is vivid dreams. The other is rapid eye movement (REM) sleep behavior disorder (RBD). Vivid dreams are drug induced, whereas RBD is due to the PD itself and often develops before PD.

VIVID DREAMS AND NIGHTMARES

Vivid dreams are a common side effect of the medications for treating PD motor symptoms. It is unknown if this is solely due to the dopamine-stimulating drugs or whether this occurs with the other PD drugs. Patients will report having dreams so realistic they may believe they really occurred. Patients may awaken in the morning and ask about the fire next door, or the barking dog down the street. In such cases the family is often extremely upset and thinks the patient has become confused or psychotic. After a few episodes, everyone recognizes the vivid dream as the explanation. In cases where the dream is quite fantastic the patient will recognize that the dream was unreal, but when the dream content is realistic, the patient may be quite confused about the dream, not being able to determine whether it was real or not.

Some books report that PD medications cause nightmares. I am unsure if this is the case. Clearly there are some patients who first develop nightmares on the PD medications, which doesn't necessarily mean the medication caused the nightmares. It is not clear that PD patients have more nightmares than other people the same age, although some texts state this as fact. I suspect that many of the cases in which nightmares surface on L-Dopa develop because the drugs make the dreams more vivid. When the dream is scary, then the realistic nature of the dream makes it a nightmare, and it becomes better remembered.

Nightmares can be a big problem for the patient and the family. As mentioned above, many PD patients vocalize in their sleep, so that they may scream during nightmares. They are also, of course, upsetting to the patient, if remembered, and if severe and frequent, may become a source of insomnia, as the patient tries to avoid sleeping. Oftentimes the patient screams and yells but later remembers nothing and seems undisturbed.

REM SLEEP BEHAVIOR DISORDER

RBD is one of the most interesting of all behavior disorders. What is astounding about it is that it is so common and so bizarre that it almost defies the imagination to realize that it was only first reported in the 1980s, despite the fact that it is a problem due to the disease itself and not to the medication treatment of PD. James Parkinson might have described it if he had learned more about the disease.

I recall thinking that it was a medication side effect, similar, perhaps, to the vivid dreams that were well known to occur with L-Dopa. REM sleep is dream sleep. About 80% of dreams occur during REM sleep. The other 20% of dreams occur without the eyes moving, and even when subjects are aroused during these dreams, the dreams are not generally recalled. These dreams are more likely to produce an emotional state rather than a typical dream. During REM sleep the normal person is "hypotonic," meaning that muscle tone is reduced. Basically, the person who is dreaming is paralyzed except for the eye movements and the muscles related to breathing. This is obviously very helpful since it would be a bad thing for people to act out their dreams while asleep.

It appears that a large percentage of PD patients, whether on medication or not, have occasional dreams during which they are not paralyzed and actually act them out. Amazingly, the dreams tend to be fairly uniform. The patient generally experiences a dream of being attacked and fighting back. This problem affects men much more than women, and the typical story is of a man dreaming of defending his wife against attack who is awakened by his wife's shrieks, as he's either punching or kicking her, or possibly trying to strangle her. This problem may predate the onset of the PD, and when RBD occurs in a middle-aged or older person, the odds are about 2:1 that PD will develop within a few years. RBD occurs only uncommonly outside of PD or related disorders.

It is usually very simple to recognize RBD, but not always. One of my patients awoke at night believing that there were intruders in the house. He saw them approach him so he jumped out the second floor window, injuring himself. Was this RBD, a nightmare that persisted for a few seconds after awakening, or was he hallucinating? I never was able to tell.

A 56-year-old normal man was sleeping soundly, then awakened due to severe pain in his mouth, finding himself on the floor in his bedroom. He had dreamed of being chased by armed men, jumped out of bed and ran into an open door, losing three teeth. Two years later he developed the first motor symptoms of PD.

A 77-year-old man punches his wife once or twice a month, and occasionally pulls her hair. When she awakens him he *describes dreams of defending her against armed intruders. When she doesn't awaken him, he recalls nothing the next morning.*

SLEEP VOCALIZATIONS

It is very common for PD patients to talk, yell, laugh, cry, and even sing in their sleep. These vocalizations are quite varied. My favorite report was of a patient who sang Italian arias when asleep. He was bilingual, having been born in Italy, but never sang English-based songs. Nor did he talk, laugh, or make other sounds.

Another interesting report was from a man who described extended one-sided conversations he heard when his wife, who had PD, was asleep. He could usually figure out what the topic was, and sometimes even who the person was. The topics were always mundane. She never revealed embarrassing secrets or said bad things about her husband. Some patients scream obscenities in their sleep despite never cursing during the day. One of my patients screams in her sleep to the point where her husband is worried the neighbors will call the police. Yet she does not describe nightmares.

In about half of cases these sounds may awaken the patient. It is unclear whether these vocalizations are made during dream sleep. It is also not clear if this is a minor form of RBD or something different. Clearly, most of the vocalizations do not reflect an angry, combative, or threatening stance, such as would be expected during a dream of being attacked, which is the usual dream in RBD. No one would expect someone to burst out into an Italian aria when threatened! Also, most of the vocalizations are not associated with major body movements such as flailing, kicking, or punching. It would probably be easier for a bed partner if RBD behavior was associated with some threatening noises so there would be a warning before the kick or punch.

Sleep vocalizations don't need to be treated unless they cause problems. Unfortunately they may cause a problem because they awaken the patient, the bed partner, or the neighbors. I am unaware of data suggesting a treatment for this, but we typically use clonazepam, the same drug that is used for RBD. There are a variety of other drugs that can be used as well.

POOR-QUALITY SLEEP

It appears that people with PD are more likely to suffer from sleep apnea than other people. The word apnea means "not breathing." Of course, if you stop breathing you die. People with sleep apnea do not die, they simply either awaken or ascend from a deep level of sleep to a lighter level. Very often they actually awaken, although they are unaware because they are awake for only seconds before falling back to sleep, descending into a deep level of sleep only to awaken in a short time because of insufficient oxygen. PD patients tend to suffer a collapse of their airway during sleep. This causes a blockage of airflow on inhaling, which is the mechanism for snoring.

Sleep apnea comes in two varieties. One is called "central sleep apnea," which refers to a syndrome in which the brain intermittently fails to generate the impulse to breathe. The patient stops breathing when in a deep sleep, and doesn't resume breathing until the blood oxygen drops to a low level. With the much more common "obstructive sleep apnea" the airways collapse and the patient begins to snore. Once the snoring begins, it increases as the depth of the breathing increases. The snoring then slowly dies down followed by a period of silence, during which there is no breathing. There is then a sudden start as the deep breathing or snoring begins anew. The apneic periods may last over 30 seconds. The patient may startle with the resumption of breathing.

In overnight sleep studies the number of awakenings may be measured and often are in the hundreds per night, sometimes a thousand or more. Some people don't sleep much more than a minute or two at a time before being awakened. These people seem to sleep like logs. They sleep ten hours at night seemingly without rousing. They awaken feeling as if they got a poor night's sleep and they are tired. They fall asleep after breakfast and are chronically sleepy. Their families make fun of them both for their snoring and for their seemingly boundless ease of falling asleep and endless need for sleep. No matter how much they sleep they're still tired, craving more.

Why people with PD are more likely than others to have sleep apnea is unknown, but it is an important consideration because it is sometimes treatable with a special mask that helps overcome the obstruction, hence restoring normal sleep without medications.

OTHER SLEEP DISORDERS

REM intrusions refer to REM, or dream sleep, developing in people who are not really asleep. They are sleepy and in the process of falling asleep or awakening. The dream plays out in their mind, but they are still somewhat conscious, in a sort of twilight state. These "intrusions," then, can be mistaken for hallucinations, delusions, or confusion. These spells need to be recognized as sleep-related problems so that antipsychotic drugs are not used inappropriately.

SLEEP "ATTACKS"

A letter to the editor of a neurology journal describing the occurrence of "sleep attacks" while driving in patients using pramipexole (Mirapex) attracted a lot of press attention. It turns out that these episodes occur with all of the dopamine agonists (Mirapex, Requip, and Neupro), but may occur in anyone who is excessively sleepy. The sleep attacks refer to sudden onset of sleep in people who later say they were not feeling particularly sleepy, so they didn't try to "fight off" the sleep onset. As a result, they got into car accidents.

However, with further evaluation, all PD patients who suffered these sleep attacks scored very high on the Epworth sleepiness scale. They all suffered from EDS. What was new was that they were unaware they were so sleepy at that particular instant. They did know that they were sleepy all the time, likely to fall asleep when standing at a red light, or when trying to read a book. This same problem occurs in all populations with EDS and not just PD patients taking dopamine agonists. This is still an important problem because PD patients who are sleepy need to be extremely cautious when driving since they may suddenly fall asleep, without the usual yawns and heavy eyelids.

An under-recognized problem is the need for excessive sleep in a small percentage of PD patients due to changes in the hypothalamus, a center deep in the brain that is important in controlling sleep. Autopsies have shown that some PD patients have changes in the same part of the brain as is affected in people with narcolepsy. There is no known connection between narcolepsy, which always begins in young people, and PD, but these PD patients develop a need for tremendous amounts of sleep and feel chronically sleepy, no matter how much good-quality sleep they get at night, or what PD medications they take during the day. It is very difficult to tease out these patients from the vast majority of PD patients who have EDS for the reasons mentioned above.

TREATMENTS

There are many approaches to treating sleep problems, but they can be extremely difficult to improve. RBD generally responds very well to low doses of clonazepam (Klonopin) given at nighttime, but clonazepam worsens balance, may contribute to confusion, and may make obstructive sleep apnea worse. While other drugs have been beneficial in RBD, the experience in using these other drugs is very limited. RLS and PLMS respond to dopamine agonists or L-Dopa, which almost all PD patients are on anyway. Sometimes it is possible to treat RLS by adjusting the medication schedule. Sleep apnea is "fixed" by special devices that force air into the lungs, but PD patients are often unable to tolerate these masks. They often feel claustrophobic or simply find the masks uncomfortable. Equally troubling are reports in medical journals that many patients with OSA, who do not have PD, don't feel any less sleepy during the day, even when their masks work! Nighttime PD medication may help someone maintain mobility so that falling asleep is easier, although this increases the risk of hallucinations or confusion during the night.

Sometimes giving a sleeping pill at night to someone who sleeps too much during the day may help restore a more normal sleep cycle. However, with the exception of RBD, the other sleep problems are often very challenging and do not always respond well to attempted treatments.

Probably the single most important approach to improving sleep habits is to address the issues of "sleep hygiene." This really is about common sense approaches, more easily suggested than implemented:

1. Limit fluids after dinner
2. No alcohol after dinner
3. Exercise regularly, but not in the evening
4. Try to go to bed and turn off the lights at about the same time each day
5. Try to get up in the morning at the same time each day
6. If napping is required, try to schedule the nap and limit its duration
7. Over time, very slowly try to reduce each nap
8. Try to schedule activities during the day that will reduce the chance of boredom or sleepiness
9. Avoid arguments or discussions of stressful things at night

No sleep medications have been tested in PD. This means, unfortunately, that there are no recommendations that can be made based on data. Different experts recommend different medications, based largely on their own personal experience with their patients.

The first question in using a medication for sleep problems is, should a sedative (sleep medication) be given to help the patient fall asleep, or should a stimulant be given in the morning to help the patient stay awake? Usually we use the sedative. Some doctors like to start with diphenhydramine (Benadryl), which is available, quite cheaply, over the counter. It is one of the ingredients in Tylenol PM. It had been used to treat PD motor symptoms, and it is usually well tolerated. One or two pills are taken at night. Benzodiazepines, a chemical class that includes diazepam (Valium), lorazepam (Ativan), alprazolam (Xanax), and temazepam (Restoril), can be very useful but contribute to imbalance and possibly confusion. All sedatives, if strong enough, may prevent a patient from awakening at night when the bladder is full, leading to urinary incontinence. This should not raise an alarm, but should trigger a reduction in the dose. Trazodone, a medication for depression and anxiety, is often used in older patients. Some doctors favor melatonin, another over-the-counter remedy that has not adequately been tested, but one study showed that 5 mg worked as well as 50, so a low dose should be tried first. Quetiapine, a very sedating antipsychotic drug, is often used in patients who need a sleep medication but are prone to hallucinations. Quetiapine may promote sleep while reducing hallucinations. Sometimes, though, it may increase confusion and contribute to lightheadedness on standing.

There's no free lunch when it comes to medications. *All* sedatives may produce side effects. But they may be worth a try because sleep problems are so troubling to patients and their families. When a PD patient gets up at night, oftentimes the spouse or caregiver does as well, leading to a very sleepy and often ornery couple.

Stimulants such as methylphenidate (Ritalin) and dextroamphetamine (Dexedrine) may be considered to keep patients awake. These are short acting, so that if taken early enough in the day they will not interfere with sleeping at night. They are contraindicated in people with uncontrolled hypertension and most heart diseases. They are drugs that some non-PD patients abuse, so that the drug must be renewed with a handwritten (not called-in or even faxed) prescription each month at the local pharmacy, not every three months via the mail. Finally, drugs such as modafinil (Provigil) and armodafinil (Nuvigil), which keep people awake without causing stimulant effects, have been tried in PD patients with mixed success. These drugs are much safer than the stimulants and should be considered. All the drugs that promote wakefulness are often restricted by insurance plans and may not be covered.

Surgery for Parkinson's Disease

Surgery for treating Parkinson's disease (PD) has made a comeback in the last 20 years. We currently use deep brain stimulation (DBS) to treat some of the motor aspects of PD in a very small percentage of patients. We have learned that this surgery sometimes produces undesirable behavioral changes. Luckily these changes are very uncommon and generally are treatable.

HISTORY

Surgery for the treatment of PD has a 60-year history. It was initially undertaken to relieve tremor in the days before computerized tomography (CT) scans. The imaging of the brain was, by current standards, not even rudimentary. To get a fix on the brain target, the patient underwent a cisternogram, which was a plain x-ray of the brain after all the spinal fluid was removed. To remove all the spinal fluid involved a spinal tap, and, with the needle still in place, strapping the patient to a chair, which was mounted on a large wheel. The wheel was rotated, with the chair fixed in its place on the wheel so that the patient was eventually turned upside down, in order to drain all the spinal fluid. This way the ventricles, which are the inner holes in the brain, fill with air, allowing them to be seen on the x-ray. This caused tremendous headaches for the patients. Unfortunately, these x-rays, primitive by current standards, did not allow the surgeon to be at all confident of where the target was. Electrical stimulation was not used. Instead a small hole was made in the brain, either by burning or freezing the tissue. The target was the thalamus, and when it worked correctly the tremor was eliminated on the opposite side. Unfortunately nothing else was helped, so patients were still slow, stooped, stiff, and walking impaired. Side effects were common and severe. L-Dopa put an end to surgery except for extreme cases of tremor.

The next popular surgery was also ablative, meaning a hole was made in the brain. Pallidotomies involved making a small hole in the globus pallidum ("pallid" for the globus pallidum and "otomy" for hole), another deep brain structure. This reduces dyskinesias and has few complications but does not help much with tremor, slowness, or gait. This has been replaced, most of the time, by our most popular current surgery, which uses continuous electrical stimulation, and also a different target, namely, the subthalamic nucleus (STN).

CURRENT SURGERY

The surgical treatment of PD has become standard, accepted therapy. It is not experimental. It is paid for by all insurance companies. It is reserved for patients who meet certain clinical criteria. It is not for most patients. The current surgery involves the insertion of a very thin wire or electrode into the STN, a location deep in the middle of the brain. The electrode is connected to a stimulator that is implanted in the chest. The wire running from the stimulator to the electrode is tunneled under the skin, up the neck and onto a wire going to the stimulator. This device is very similar to a cardiac pacemaker, the main difference being that the DBS stimulates the brain rather than the heart. From the outside they look the same.

Although most electrode targets are the STN, some patients have their electrode placed in another location, the globus pallidum (GP). The GP is another deep brain structure, which is considerably larger and therefore easier to hit than the STN. It is less effective against slowness but more effective against dyskinesias. After GP surgery the anti-PD medications are usually not much altered, whereas after the STN surgery the doses are generally quite a bit lower. Behavioral complications are almost entirely limited to STN stimulation. There have been very few behavioral complications with GP stimulation. These problems include anxiety, apathy, cognitive decline, hallucinations, and mania. The benefits of STN over GP stimulation are widely believed but not yet supported by hard evidence. Sometimes, when tremor is the only PD problem, and is not responsive to medication, the target is the thalamus, but this is uncommon.

DBS does not "cure" PD. It is, however, very effective for stopping severe tremors that do not respond to L-Dopa or any of the PD medications, and is also very helpful for eliminating clinical fluctuations that are otherwise uncontrollable. It works especially well in younger patients who have bothersome dyskinesias when they're "on" and problems with mobility when they're "off." The DBS eliminates the fluctuations and usually the dyskinesias as well. Most patients can reduce their PD medications and occasional patients can actually stop their PD drugs entirely. The general outcome, when the procedure goes well, is to make the patient function at his best level on PD medication, all day, without fluctuations or dyskinesias. In other words, the patient will not usually improve beyond his best presurgical state, but the "off" period problems will be eliminated and the patient will be at his "best" all day, every day. Thus, if a patient can't walk despite the best medical treatment, then DBS will not restore the ability to walk. If the patient can walk for a half-hour each day, but the rest of the day is either incapacitated by immobility or severe dyskinesias, then the surgery may work wonders, rendering the patient mobile the whole day, without the disabling dyskinesias. And not only will the patient be better, but he will be on less medication as well, with fewer side effects.

The treatment with DBS takes place in two stages. The first stage involves the placement of the electrode. In other words, the wire that will deliver the small electrical charges is inserted into the brain at one end and attached to the skull at the other. The wire is then connected to the stimulator, which is implanted under the skin, usually in the chest. Although the stimulator is tested in the operating room, it is then turned off. The stimulator is usually not turned on for treatment until about two weeks after the wire is implanted. Sometimes, when a stimulator wire is implanted on each side, the procedures may be performed one or two weeks apart, so that the stimulators aren't turned on for treatment until about two weeks after the second stimulator is implanted.

Sometimes the patients have changes immediately after the operation, even though the stimulator hasn't been turned on. Why should this happen if the stimulator isn't turned on? The wire, although quite fine, still produces some brain damage and therefore works just like the old-time surgery. In the days before DBS, the operation for PD involved making a hole in a part of the brain. No one made these holes, called "ablations," in the STN because we were afraid that it would cause another severe movement disorder called hemiballism (in which patients have violent, flailing movements of an arm or leg). With the electrical stimulation, the size of the stimulation became adjustable, so that excessive movements can be limited by a reduction in the stimulation. When the wire is inserted into the STN, a small amount of damage is done, and some swelling, called edema, develops. In most patients this isn't enough to cause problems or to change anything, but in some it is, and they come out of the operating room much improved. This has been called "the microelectrode effect," as it is thought due to the microelectrode causing minor damage to the STN.

BEHAVIORAL ASPECTS

The major contraindications for surgery are cognitive and behavioral. Although the surgery does not reduce intellectual function in normal people, it appears to cause significant worsening in patients with mild dementia or psychotic symptoms. Most centers, therefore, obtain neuropsychological evaluations before scheduling the surgery. Brain surgery can alter behavior, but not usually.

It was a great surprise, when the procedures were first being done, that patients occasionally had very peculiar behavioral responses to the operation or to the stimulation. No one had ever done surgery in this region of the brain before, unless there was an abscess or tumor. People have all sorts of unexpected behaviors after a brain operation. There is such tremendous psychic stress before the operation—fear about a bad outcome, fear about a disappointing improvement—that there may be a great relief when the operation is over. Although the patient isn't unconscious during the procedure, drugs to control anxiety are used, and these can produce behavioral changes. The PD medications are also altered for the operation so the combination of stress and changed medications that work on the brain, and even the change in the environment, may cause someone to develop weird behaviors. However, with experience, it has become clear that the behavioral alterations we see are actually a direct result of the small damage done to the brain.

An important paper published in the *New England Journal of Medicine* described a PD patient who became extremely depressed when the DBS settings were changed. This patient had no history of depression, and the feelings of overwhelming sadness and loss of interest in living had developed over seconds. And they resolved within seconds of the stimulator being turned off. This was an astounding observation for at least two reasons. One was that it clearly demonstrated the "mind–brain" connection and that minor changes even in tiny parts of the brain can produce major alterations. The other was that this tiny collection of brain cells, far away from the parts of the brain that neuroscientists had thought were the important parts of the brain for behavior, mood, and thinking, was integrally involved. There had probably never been such a clear demonstration that depression was not that much different than arm or leg movements, that parts of the brain were responsible for different behaviors including movements, sensations, memory, language, and even emotions. Emotion comes from the brain and brain disorders alter emotions. It seems as simple and obvious as "ABC" but isn't because emotions are so multifaceted.

Long-term studies on DBS outcomes have shown that neuropsychological testing has been quite stable. There is very little change over time, and this is likely due to aging and the natural course of the disease.

In general, cognition does not change. However, certain outcomes look as if they may be the result of surgery. For example, a few suicide attempts and completions have been ascribed to DBS. Suicide is an extremely uncommon event in PD patients otherwise. Why this is so remains unclear. As far as I know, I've had one patient attempt and commit suicide in over 30 years of practice. A single suicide in any group, while cause for concern, would not alarm many people, but several attempts suggest a relationship to the surgery. It is not generally believed that the suicides were due to disappointment with the surgical outcome. Suicide, while generally thought to reflect depression, doesn't always. Sometimes it occurs because of impulsive behavior and may represent anger or frustration in someone who becomes impulsive. Most likely the suicides were due to an increase in impulsivity.

Probably the most difficult problem in DBS patients is depression in someone with a good motor response to the surgery.

In one paper, the authors observed that, "one of the most intriguing symptoms observed after surgery was apathy ... which often is expressed as a fatigue by the patient." This was very unexpected as the patients should be moving faster and more easily. There was an unexpected conflict in outcomes, which pointed to an important effect on behavioral perception. These apathetic patients are not demented or depressed, conditions with which apathy is frequently associated. The authors of this article consider the apathy a form of "loss of psychic self-motivation." The patients describe feeling too tired to begin any activity yet will undertake jobs they are ordered to do, and later report enjoying the performance of the activity. They are amotivational, although they may have plans for numerous activities. They may require someone to program and ignite them, like an explosive without a detonator. Loss of initiative is, of course, a common problem in PD, so surgery that alters the circuits of the brain involving PD motor activity, not surprisingly, also alters behavior in a way that is consistent with behavior problems in PD.

Depression improves to a small degree with the surgery. However, some people become depressed from the surgery or the stimulation, as mentioned above. The depression is highly variable, from the overwhelming, sudden onset with a change in stimulator settings, to the case, as described in the vignette below, where the connection to the stimulator isn't clear.

In one case at our center a patient never commented on depression. However, when she came in for one visit and her stimulator was changed, she suddenly commented that she felt much better. Her motor function hadn't changed much but she said she felt like a heavy weight had been lifted from her shoulders, that ever since the stimulator had been first turned on she had felt mildly to moderately depressed, but since the onset wasn't sudden and the sadness wasn't overwhelming she didn't connect her mood change to the stimulator.

Hypomania, that is, a mild form of mania, may occur. This almost always occurs within the first three months of surgery. Hypomania is characterized primarily by an elated mood. Patients feel excessively well, optimistic, and expansive. They may need less sleep than they used to, get more pleasure out of everything that they do, feel more powerful, more in control and confident. Unfortunately, while they feel well and radiate self-satisfaction, it may be very incongruent to their situation. They may need a lot of help but deny their need. They may become inappropriately sexual or develop marked increases in sexual needs. In one of my patients with manic-depression and PD the better she felt the more I worried about her mental illness. Her PD was sufficiently advanced that she should be having problems due to her limitations, so if she reported that things were "terrific," I knew the mania was setting in.

Mania is the most common problem I've seen with DBS, but it has been entirely controllable except for our patient with the manic-depressive disorder. In fact, the operation was refused at one center because of this problem, but performed at another with full awareness of the possible aftereffects. Ultimately, our patient did very well.

Two patients experienced transient episodes, early after surgery, of aggressive and impulsive behavior.

Psychosis occurred in four patients. In two of these patients dementia was present. In another the psychosis was long-lasting. Since psychosis may occur in any PD patient on medications, the only thing that can definitively link the stimulation to the psychosis is the occurrence of psychotic symptoms with the stimulator turned on and resolution with the stimulator turned off. It was not clear in this report whether the psychosis remitted off the stimulation. My own experience, with a patient who became psychotic for the first time after the stimulation was begun, is that her psychosis continued to worsen even after the stimulator was turned off. At autopsy it turned out that she had developed dementia with Lewy bodies as well as Alzheimer's disease. At the time of the surgery her neuropsychological examination revealed no evidence of dementia.

In our center, a patient with a long history of manic depression became severely manic immediately on return from the operating room. She accused a male staff member of rape, and other staff members of trying to poison her or do other bad things. She hallucinated and tried to escape from the hospital. This lasted about five days before she became her usual self. She remembered the episode as extremely unpleasant.

Another report described several days of delirium immediately after the operation. Anxiety, cognitive decline, and even hallucinations have been reported after STN lead placement. In occasional cases the changes were permanent.

One problem that a patient at our center encountered was an increase in cross-dressing. The patient had crossed-dressed for many years, before his PD developed, but after his DBS surgery this increased. He was less inhibited than he had been before the surgery.

In general, if a patient with PD develops a behavior problem within a short time of a stimulator adjustment, and if a readjustment of the stimulator produces a reversion of the abnormal behavior, it is safe to assume that the stimulation caused the behavior. But if a problem develops during the course of chronic stimulation and does not change with discontinuation of the stimulation, then it makes more sense, I believe, to blame the abnormal behavior on the disease process itself or the medications, but not the stimulation. So far as is known, DBS does not produce long-standing changes.

See Appendix A, "Winning the Battle but Losing the War."

14

. . . .

Driving

Driving is a contentious issue in Parkinson's disease (PD). Many patients can continue to drive safely, but not all. Reaction time is slowed, and recent studies show that PD patients are less adept at scanning the environment and tend to miss more signs and other visual images than others. The question arises frequently as to when the line from being safe to unsafe is being crossed. There is no good way short of a driving test to decide who should be able to continue to drive. I always recommend that an impartial driving professional make the decision based on an on-road driving evaluation.

Driving is perhaps the single most difficult issue for doctors and families in the management of PD. Doctors are not very good at assessing who can or cannot drive safely, and there are few of us who would perform a road test with one of our suspect patients.

In some respects, the issue of driving can be finessed. When I tell a patient I think they should give up driving, the usual response is, "I've been driving for 55 years and haven't been in an accident in the last 25. I'm a safe driver and could teach you a thing or two about driving safety. When I can't drive safely, I'll stop driving."

The problem is that people who drive unsafely think that all the problems are due to the other drivers. Lack of safety is usually due to lack of insight. The patient who reacts too slowly or fails to heed all the stop and yield signs, or who stays too far to the left or the right of the lane, always does so unknowingly. If they knew they were not driving well they would either improve their driving or stop driving.

So, how do I finesse this? I tell the patient that I can't really assess their driving skills accurately. The patient may be capable of winning the Indianapolis 500 for all I know, but my job is to protect both them and the public, and if I think they might be unsafe then I have an obligation to tell them my opinion. I point out that I cannot force them to stop driving, although in some states the doctor is required to report medically unsafe drivers to the department of motor vehicles. I therefore tell them that they can "prove" their driving safety by taking a road test. In Rhode Island, there are two ways to do this, and this is probably true throughout the country. They can give up their license and take the state licensing exam again. If they pass then they can drive. An alternative is to take a road test at a private driving school that offers this service. I don't know how common this is, but it is available in my home state.

A *65-year-old woman can barely walk due to freezing gait. In fact, she can hardly move her feet even when she's sitting. In addition to that she has a severe language problem. She can't say what she wants to all the time, and has difficulty reading.*

I tell her that she can't drive because she can't move her feet. She tells me that she's a first-rate driver and is very safe. I challenge her to give up her license and take the tests again. She returns three months later, triumphant. She took the test and passed. It was inconceivable to me that she could pass, but she did.

*A*n 80-year-old man with moderately advanced Alzheimer's disease (AD) was told by his doctor that he couldn't drive anymore. The man protested but the family was greatly relieved. They had driven with him or seen him drive and had asked him to stop. He was not allowed to drive any grandchildren and no one would drive with him. He took his driving test and passed, much to everyone's amazement. His daughter reported that at the end of the driving test, he left the car while it was still in "drive," so that the car started moving down the street without any driver. Although the examiner witnessed this, the patient was still given a passing grade.

*A*one-eyed patient took the vision exam and failed, so he was asked to repeat the exam, again and again, until he passed on the fourth try. He subsequently received his driving approval.

How can one assess the issue of driving safety? Driving is terribly important to so many people. While most people would like the idea of having a chauffeur, few of us want it forced upon us, especially men. Driving has both real, tangible meaning and deeply symbolic implications. Giving up driving is, for many patients, the giving up of independence. Even though the patient may not have driven in the past two years, the notion that he will never drive again often makes the patient desperate. "What if my wife has a heart attack and I have to drive her to the hospital?" "What if I have to get a medicine at the drug store, which is a mile away?" "What if...?" I have patients who have agreed not to drive but nevertheless still refuse to give up their car. It is too important a symbol of independence to them.

There have been a few studies of driving and PD. There are several aspects of PD that may interfere with good driving skills. The first is bradykinesia, or slowness. The PD patient is slow performing most tasks and may react to emergency situations more slowly than a normal person. This clearly is a potential problem.

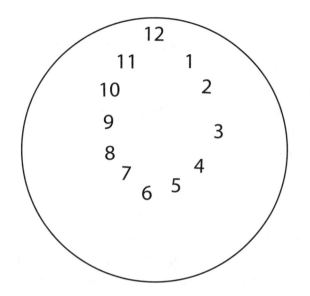

Secondly, and this is something that most PD patients and their families don't consider, PD patients frequently have a problem with visual–spatial orientation (see Chapter 17). This is the way that people judge their environment. In one of the simplest of examples, if one asks a PD patient to draw the numbers of a clock in a circle, in most cases there will be a fairly stereotypic "halo" around the numbers. The 12 is entered correctly but the 1, 2, and 3 are put a bit close together so that the three is not one-fourth of the way around the circle. In addition, there is room between the numbers and the circle itself. The remaining numbers are then entered with a large space at the bottom between the 6 and the circle's bottom. The numbers are too close together, and there is a circle of space, or halo, between the numbers and the circle itself. This is not a big deal. It is only illustrative of the problem, which is that PD patients do not interpret their geometric world with the same geometry as the rest of us.

A much less common—but still common enough—problem, is that of misjudging where a seat is. Some PD patients will attempt to sit down when the chair is not at the proper distance from their bottom, so that the patient places only half of their backside on the chair, sometimes not even that, causing a fall. Or the patient can't judge the height of the seat and plops down into the chair, occasionally causing it to fall over backwards, with the patient in the chair. These problems simply illustrate the potential problem in judging distances, an obvious necessity in driving. These patients often drive too far to one side of the road.

Another problem that perhaps drew the most attention to driving in PD was a report from Columbia University describing so-called sleep attacks in PD (see Chapter 12). This report, which was widely published in American and international newspapers, sparked a large series of studies looking primarily at sleepiness in PD, but also a few driving studies. What I believe has emerged as a consensus opinion is that all of the dopamine agonists (pramipexole, ropinerole, rotigotine, and probably bromocriptine) produce sleepiness. However, as noted in Chapter 12, PD patients have many reasons for excessive sleepiness, which may have nothing to do with dopamine agonists or other medications. People who are excessively sleepy sometimes fall asleep suddenly and have no recollection of having been sleepy before falling asleep. These are "sleep attacks." When the Columbia group described them initially, they had detected the problem only in drivers who had fallen asleep while driving, but that's largely because these patients had accidents. People who fall asleep driving but wake up before the accident are unlikely to report this to their doctor, and people who fall asleep suddenly while watching TV or reading the newspaper are also unlikely to describe this as a problem. These "sleep attacks" virtually never occur in people who are not sleepy. Thus, a major risk factor for car accidents is sleepiness during the day.

A *56-year-old patient with PD taking pramipexole and benztropine for his PD was involved in a car accident in which he ran a red light and hit another car. Luckily no one was injured. He told the policeman that he failed to respond in time so the policeman reported him to the motor vehicle department which removed his license.*

He told me a different story. He told me that he had fallen asleep, awaking on impact. He had been afraid to tell the policeman, assuming that it was safer in some way to tell him the problem was his PD. I suspect that he made a mistake in that decision. I think the policeman would have been inclined to assume that anyone can fall asleep driving, but that slowed reaction time is a definite problem that isn't a one-time issue for someone with PD.

The most dangerous problem for drivers is dementia. Demented patients are the ones most likely to get into accidents because they usually lack insight. The average PD patient knows that his driving skills are not what they once were. He will continue to drive but will usually limit himself to the safest situations, rarely taking any risks. These patients drive during the day only, on streets they know very well, in areas and times where there is little traffic, and only when the weather is good. No snow, rain, ice, and so on.

The single most difficult driving problem for elderly patients is turning left onto a two-way road. This requires the ability to judge oncoming traffic from both directions, as well as to merge into a lane at an appropriate speed.

It is common for all of us to occasionally "forget" where we are or take a wrong turn because we're daydreaming while driving. For a demented patient this can be the kiss of death. Once they feel a little disoriented they may become increasingly disoriented, which usually brings with it anxiety and increasingly impaired judgment. Anxiety causes people to make bad decisions. Anxiety in demented people simply exacerbates an already bad situation.

There are a variety of driving "tests" for PD patients. Some of these are computerized and involve a patient basically playing a video game, having to react to unexpected situations, or expected disruptions: a ball bounces in front of the car, suggesting the possibility of a child appearing in a second or two in hot pursuit; a man riding a bicycle may suddenly veer into the lane; a car in front may stop suddenly, causing a rear-end fender-bender if the reaction is delayed. But no computer test is as reliable as real-life testing. At some point there is likely to be a computer test that exactly simulates road testing, just as there are good pilot simulators for airplane pilots and astronauts, but so far no such simulator is in use.

A 2005 study from England found that more than 50% of PD patients who volunteered to be in a driving study would not have passed an official state-run driving test. These patients had all attended lectures on driving safety in PD and can be assumed to represent the PD patients *least* likely to have driving problems. One of the very important results of the study was the poor correlation between the driving instructor's view on the patient's safety and the patient's own assessment of his driving skills. The study concluded that driving safety could not be inferred from the driver's own assessment or from the motor examination in the office. An editorial accompanying the article suggested that "slowness of movement and reaction time are likely to play important roles in driving performance, but that other factors, such as impaired visual–spatial processing, planning, and sequencing are also likely to contribute to the difficulties."

The family often precipitates a discussion of driving capabilities. It is rare, in my experience, for the family to argue with me about driving. Probably half the time, it is the family that approaches me, in private, telling me that the PD patient should not be driving. The family is often afraid to discuss this openly because it will provoke anger in the patient and hostility toward the family member who brought it up. It becomes the doctor's role then to bring this topic up and to take responsibility, defusing a potentially very harmful situation at home. Whenever a family member tells me in private that the patient is a risky driver, I assume they are correct. At some point during my evaluation I bring up the topic of driving and ask if the patient drives. The answer is generally, "Yes, but only a little bit. I'm very safe." I often then suggest that the person get a professional assessment, with all sides agreeing to honor the outcome.

I developed a talk that I give to patients who I counsel not to drive.

"I know that what I'm about to say is going to upset you and I also know that you are going to disagree with me, but it's my responsibility to tell you that I think you may be an unsafe driver. I'm sure you think

I'm wrong. If you agreed with me you wouldn't be driving at all. And you also know that I've never seen you drive, so what I'm telling you is what I think, not what I know. But my job is to be fair and honest and to try to keep you and others safe. If you get into a car accident that I might have prevented, then some of the responsibility is mine. I'm sure you understand this. I want you to understand that it's very difficult for me to ask you not to drive. I fully understand how important driving is in our society, and that your lifestyle may change dramatically as a result of your stopping driving. I know that driving helps make you independent and that PD makes you increasingly dependent, so that giving up driving is another blow against your independence.

"I'm going to tell you what I tell all my patients who I tell not to drive. Imagine that you're driving down a street and a small child runs in front of your car so that you hit her. It may have been the case that no driver could have avoided hitting the child, that the accident was clearly 100% the child's fault. Unfortunately, there won't be any slow-motion replays like there are on TV. If your son or daughter was driving, everyone would yell at the child or the parent for letting the child run unsupervised in front of the car. But when you get out of the car, everyone is going to say, 'Why is this old person with PD driving? He's a danger. Look what he did to this little kid. He should have known better.' The same accident, but with different drivers, will, I believe, produce two different interpretations. In one case witnesses will blame the child and in the other they will blame the driver, especially if he's old and has PD. Not only that, but you yourself will think it's your fault. You'll say, 'I should have listened to the doctor, to my family. Maybe they were right. Now look at what I've done.' And there will be no way to replay the situation, to assign blame. No one will ever know who's to blame, and once the damage is done it is too late. You need to think about this before you decide to continue driving. Think about how you'd feel if this happened to your grandchild.

"But if you don't agree with me, and I'm sure I'm not completely accurate in deciding who's a safe or unsafe driver, then take a driving test. You can give up your driver's license and take the test again, or you can hire a driving school to take you out on a road test. If you pass then you can continue driving and if you fail you have to stop."

There are patients who I think can drive safely but in limited circumstances. In most states there is no "limited license" except for people with a driver's permit or a probationary license. For learners in some states, or newly licensed drivers, it is illegal to drive during certain hours, or to transport more than one minor at a time. I often tell people that they should restrict their driving to light traffic areas, well-known routes, daylight hours, good weather, easy parking, low probability of children playing. They should avoid highways for obvious reasons.

A clever study had PD and age-matched, non-PD drivers comment to a researcher in the car every time they passed a restaurant or a blinking yellow light. The PD patients missed a substantial portion of both compared to the non-PD patient, indicating that the PD drivers didn't notice things as well as the non-PD drivers. Almost all accidents occur due to something unexpected happening. In PD, more unexpected things are likely to occur due to the problem of not noticing everything that is in the environment.

From the same 2005 study out of England mentioned earlier: "Drivers with PD were rated as significantly less safe than controls, and more than half of the drivers with PD would not have passed a state-based driving test. The driver safety ratings were more strongly related to disease duration than to their 'on' time Unified Parkinson's Disease Rating Scale (UPDRS). Drivers with PD made significantly more errors than the control group during maneuvers that involved changing lanes and lane keeping, monitoring their blind spot, reversing, car parking, and traffic light controlled intersections."

15

. . . .

Caregivers and Family

People who live with or provide care for those with Parkinson's disease (PD) are often crucially important for the well-being of the patient. Doctors too often focus on the patient and the specific PD-related problems and lose track of the whole picture, how the patient and the family is doing. It is important to check on the caregiver as well as the patient. The health and well-being of the caregiver may be just as important for the patient as attending to the patient's own problems.

Not all PD patients have family members or friends who would be classified as caregivers, but most probably do. Health professionals don't think of the "caregiver" as the person who necessarily provides all the care. Rather, I believe that doctors and the medical community think of caregivers as people who provide some care, but also have responsibility for helping out if and when things go wrong. Perhaps more importantly, not all who are classified as "caregivers" consider themselves in that category. Many are simply caring spouses, family members, and friends who help out as needed, just as the patient has and may continue to help them as well. The term "caregiver" implies that the PD patient is always needing and receiving some sort of care. This is certainly not true, but many do, in fact, need and receive this care, and the caregiver is definitely part of the social constellation. For those who are involved, but not providing services, the future often carries the risk of increasing involvement and need.

Many PD patients live on their own. They work full-time jobs, maintain households, and do all the work that needs to be done. But this is not always the case, and, after a period of years, is rarely the case. PD puts a major crimp in one's lifestyle. Unfortunately PD patients who do not have people they can rely upon for help often end up in nursing homes.

A popular book that analyzed changing lifestyles in America was called *Bowling Alone*. It described a major change in which membership in groups and group activities had been declining in the United States for many years. People were less likely to join community bowling teams, hence the book's title. They were less likely to be in church groups, or to participate in other group activities. This tendency toward isolation works against those who become ill because illness increases isolation, and isolation increases the burden of illness.

The reason for having a special chapter for caregivers is that they are too often excluded from our analyses of what's going on in the patient's life. And, I suspect, they are the majority of who actually reads this book. One of the most important lessons I ever learned about treating the "whole patient" was from a psychiatrist. He was a very smart, overconfident, and unpleasant fellow, due to his arrogance, but he taught me something crucial when he treated a patient with PD who we shared. He told me that treating the wife of the patient for *her* depression was what needed to be done. And he was correct. She was constantly crying, bemoaning the fate of her husband, struck down by PD at the age of 78, and complaining about all the things he couldn't do anymore. She was more bothered by his limitations than he was. When she was treated for her depression, life improved for both of them.

This anecdote drove home to me the truth of the teaching that one doesn't treat a patient, one treats a family. This can be a difficult situation for a number of reasons. The main problem is that only the patient is actually my patient. The spouse, the children, the significant others are not my patients. In fact, with the federal Health Insurance Portability and Accountability Act guidelines, I can't even discuss the patient (legally) with interested family members without a release from the patient.

A *middle-aged woman who has had PD for 10 years complained to me every meeting for over three years about the lack of understanding and appreciation for her illness that she got at home. Her husband, she reported, won't accompany her to doctor visits, even if she asks him to. He apparently cuts her no slack at home and blames her for the children's underperformance in school and at work. He accompanied her to a single doctor's appointment, when they went for a second opinion to see someone famous. At this meeting the doctor openly blamed the husband for the patient's miseries, and decried his lack of sympathy and understanding. Rather than feeling guilty or talking about reconciliation, the husband vowed to never see that "crock" again, or to visit another doctor with her again.*

So what can I do when I learn that they have already failed out of marriage counseling? The answer is, precious little. After several years, I finally met the man. We discussed the patient's situation, and to a much more limited extent, the home situation. I suggested another trial of marriage counseling, but I was skeptical that it would, in fact, be helpful. He wasn't a caregiver but his attitude was a significant cause for the patient's distress.

For each problem that the patient has, problems that the caregiver, particularly the spouse, has, magnify each one. There have been studies of caregiver stress but doctors frequently don't pay much attention. Many of these are published in the nursing journals, as if this is purely a "nursing" or "women's" issue. We know that hallucinations are very stressful for the caregiver, perhaps more so than for the patient, but we don't know how often depression in the PD patient is associated with depression in the caregivers or other family members. It is easy to imagine that the caregiver's depression induces the PD patient's depression or vice versa. It is also easy to imagine that if the caregiver is chronically anxious, the patient will become increasingly anxious as well.

In general, it is a good idea to consider the whole family and social constellation. Doing so, though, is practically impossible, at least for the doctor or nurse practitioner. If the family can be referred to a family counselor, usually a social worker, who is used to dealing with whole constellations that center around chronic disease, then the chance of achieving some meaningful improvements is possible.

In a study published in 2006, an English group surveyed 123 caregivers using a mailed questionnaire. What they found will not surprise anyone, but does drive home the point that even when problems are obvious, they may not be getting the attention they deserve.

Over 40% of caregivers thought that their own health had suffered as a result of their partner's PD. About half suffered from depression. As would be anticipated, the likelihood of the caregiver's being depressed correlated with how long the patient had PD. It also correlated with the patient's level of depression as well. The caregiver's and patient's quality of life were closely intertwined. The most stressful aspects of the illness for the caregiver were the behavioral problems of the patient. Falls and physical dysfunction were very important too, but this study underscored observations from other studies in the United States that caregiver burden as well as risk of nursing home placement was more closely linked to psychiatric problems associated with the PD than with the movement disorder aspects of PD.

Treating caregivers of PD patients has been modeled on treatment of caregivers in Alzheimer's and other diseases. A popular form of talk therapy called CBT or cognitive behavioral therapy was found to be helpful. CBT "seeks to develop both cognitive and behavioral skills to cope with current stressors, making it particularly suitable to the complex demands and stresses of the caregiving role." CBT improved quality of life as well as reduced caregiver strain and sense of burden.

Interestingly, children of PD patients fare better than caregivers. In a study of adolescent and adult children of PD patients (one-third of subjects were between 12 and 24, the rest were older), who were not caregivers, only 17% were depressed, as compared with 50% of caregivers. Quality of life of the children was adversely affected by their parent's PD. The children reported less family cohesiveness than families without a PD patient. The children reported "an impact on familial communication and functioning, their own development, hopes and plans, their emotional well-being, attitudes and outlook on the future, and the social support they receive." Younger children were more likely than older ones to feel embarrassed by the illness, thus implying a negative effect on socialization. The children generally thought that if they had more information on PD that coping and adjustment would be easier.

At a time when doctors are actually having their reimbursements *reduced* for seeing elderly patients in the United States it is hard to expect them to be especially keen to take on family problems in addition to coping with their actual patient. However, the patient's "illness," the pathological entity we call PD, unfortunately has a large ripple effect. But the family is not an ocean; the ripple doesn't fade away to nothingness. The family is a limited unit. This ripple occurs in a container. The ripples are reflected off the sides and come back. Sometimes these ripples build up and overwhelm the patient and the family. The smaller the family, the greater the ripple builds up. What's good for the family is usually what's good for the patient.

It's always good to have family members present at the doctor visits. The caregiver and the rest of the family not only provide another point of view on the patient's illness but also may reveal the strains in the family unit.

Since this book is for patients and their families and friends, not for doctors, it is not appropriate, perhaps, to point out the need to address family and caregiver needs and concerns. However, I do think it helpful for the family to describe their own needs and problems. The patient does not need to be the center of every discussion. It helps for the doctor to understand the environment at home as treating the patient may involve treating someone else. It may be very useful for the caregiver to discuss these problems with his or her own primary care doctor, or to seek psychological support. In most cases, the first place to look for succor is with a local PD support group, many of which have caregiver meetings. At these meetings, the patients are not allowed so that honest discussions may be held.

There are so many gigantic problems for caregivers that I cannot single out one as the most important. For many caregivers, the issue of nursing home placement is always in the background. Spouses or children often promise their loved one that they'll never go to a nursing home unless they want to. But sometimes it is, in fact, required. A broken caregiver is not useful to the patient. How many petite 80-year-old women are caring for their 200-pound husbands who can't get in or out of bed, fall down once a week and have to call the rescue service to pick him up? What happens when the sole caregiver gets sick? Oftentimes the PD patient refuses to consider a nursing home, preferring to spend the day at home, watching TV and falling asleep, a prisoner. It would be dishonest of me to say that nursing homes are always wonderful places. But some are very nice, and many patients and families, including patients who refused to consider one, are happily surprised by a smooth transition. At a good nursing home the care is reliable, the people nice, and several good outcomes may develop: new friends, frequent activities to engage the mind, the body and social skills, and a release from the guilt of making the caregiver one's slave. The caregiver may experience the relief of no longer having to worry about the next fall, getting the patient to the bathroom, or injuring her back. And nursing homes are not prisons. If you don't like it, you can move out or transfer to another.

There have been studies of caregiver stress and caregiver burden in PD. Some interesting findings are that stress is greater for younger caregivers than older, presumably related to the younger having conflicting duties, caring for their own children, working, and so on, which older, retired, spouses don't have. Another interesting issue is the stress that arises from worrying about the patient. One American study found that the stress of worrying about patient safety outweighed the stress of worrying about physical issues such as getting the patient in and out of the bath or the bed. Several reports have shown that the stress of dealing with a mentally impaired patient is much greater than dealing with a physically impaired patient, so that it is easier on the caregiver to help a PD patient who needs a walker but is mentally competent than to care for one who is able to walk without difficulty but is demented or having psychotic symptoms. This is reflected in the fact that caregiver stress is greater in those caring for people with Alzheimer's disease (AD) than it is for people with PD.

I should note that my comments about caregiving reflect my own perceptions and those in the literature concerning American and western European cultures. The stresses, supports, and expectations may be quite different in other cultures.

A less cataclysmic but more common problem is setting limits. It is very difficult to determine where to draw the line between "tough love" and insensitivity. When the PD patient is constantly asking for help with chores he can easily do himself, it is natural to refuse to help, but PD patients can usually do most things for themselves. The issue is how much time it requires, and how hard it is. Yes, the patient can put on her dress by herself but it may take several minutes. Maybe she can put her bra on most of the time, but perhaps not always, depending on the bra. Will it be "babying" by helping too much? Will too much helping simply lead to increased dependence, converting the caregiver to slave status? I am rarely comfortable giving advice to families coping with these issues. I usually validate the problem, pointing out both sides to the discussion and encouraging them to work out solutions, knowing that there will be no "correct" solution. Some patients take pride in not involving a caregiver with getting dressed, for example, while others are angry that they have to take 15 minutes to get on their shirt and then they're told that they've done the buttons incorrectly.

This brings up the issue of nagging, which I've addressed in Appendix E. I have come to the conclusion that nagging is okay for two situations, safety and exercise. Certainly there may be other situations where nagging is needed, but overall, it is OK to nag the patient to use the walker or cane if that's required to reduce the risk of falling, and exercise, which is probably the most important thing a patient can do to slow motor symptom progression.

An issue that drives caregivers crazy is the overdependence that sometimes develops, to the point where a caregiver cannot be out of eyesight of the patient. Even going to the bathroom may require reassurance that the patient isn't being abandoned, and the idea of going out to run chores alone creates a catastrophe rivaled by sending one's child off to school for the first time. And there are clear parallels, despite the differences in ages. Sometimes the PD patient needs to be treated like a small child if he behaves like one. This outcome, which is fairly common, is a good reason why the topic addressed above, of where to draw the line between "tough love" and "babying," is so important. We all fear that "babying" may lead to overdependence so that the patient cannot function on his own, or even be left alone, even in "safe" situations. As with all problems, an ounce of prevention is worth a pound of cure, so as this situation evolves, and it rarely develops suddenly (although it may after a serious illness in a caregiver), it is important to try to set up regular routines. It is particularly helpful to insist on participation at a senior day care facility at least half a day each week, with the goal of slow increases. This not only enriches the life of the patient, but frees up the caregivers as well. Sometimes it takes a fight to do it, and, just like dropping the child off at school, often gets easier each time, until it becomes something the patient may even look forward to.

An occasional issue with caregivers arises when the caregivers are the children. Very often the work gets apportioned very unevenly.

First of all women seem to do most of the work in most families. There seems to be an unspoken rule that this type of care is women's work, so that women often feel guilty if they don't do it, and the men feel like their sisters and wives are "supposed" to do it. Secondly, it is common for one child to live closer, often much closer, to the patient, making it "natural" for that person to supply more of the care. Thirdly, a particularly devastating problem is the child who lives far enough away that he cannot supply any help other than money and moral support, yet acts as the "moral overseer," telling the local children that they're not doing enough, provoking guilt but without bearing any responsibility. The most common scenarios involve sons who moved far away and daughters who live nearby. The daughter does the work, often at great expense to her own family, and reaps the reward of her brother telling her that she's not doing a good job, particularly if the PD patient complains, pitting one child against the other. However, there are many scenarios, and as Tolstoy pointed out in *Anna Karenina*, each family is unhappy in its own way. The reason I'm writing this is that these issues are best addressed consciously. The doctor can only help the family understand the dynamic, and even then, not much since doctor visits have such limited time allotments.

PD PATIENT AS CAREGIVER

Some PD patients are themselves caregivers. Many of my patients are caregivers to their elderly parents. Some need to help their children, usually financially or with providing housing. A few of my PD patients provide care for their adult, disabled children, and, as with all people with such responsibilities, have to worry about the impact PD progression will have on their own ability to provide care to others.

16

. . . .

Electroconvulsive Therapy

I briefly touched on electroconvulsive therapy (ECT) in the chapter on depression but would like to give it a bit more exposure because it is a useful treatment that is too often overlooked. ECT would seem like an unattractive treatment for anything. It is an epileptic seizure induced by passing a strong electric current into the brain. In general, neurologists try to prevent seizures.

Many years ago psychiatrists noted that some of their patients, with a wide variety of psychiatric disorders, experienced transient improvement in their behavioral problems after they had suffered an epileptic seizure. In these patients, the seizures were natural, occurring as the result of brain disorders such as old strokes, tumors, old brain injuries, new brain injuries, or inherited seizure conditions. Since there was so little to offer in the way of treatment for the seriously mentally ill, and much of it in the early twentieth century seems in retrospect to have been more punishment than therapy, any opportunity to improve a mental illness generated interest. The first approach to generating seizures was to give insulin, which produced a massive drop in blood sugar, which would produce a generalized epileptic fit in many, although not all, people. For any who have seen a convulsive seizure, this is a scary business. Muscles stiffen to a degree that is not possible while conscious. Patients often have tremendous muscle spasms and injure themselves. Afterwards they are profoundly tired, often confused and go to sleep for hours. Unfortunately, the psychiatric problems that improved with seizures generally required several seizures. This was a gruesome process. And, of course, no one had a clue as to how it worked, and, at the beginning, no one really knew who would benefit.

With time and research, vast improvements have been made in the administration of the seizure. A brain seizure is still required, but with modern anesthetics, it is no longer a scary business. Patients are sedated and once asleep are briefly paralyzed while the electric shock is applied to the scalp. This shock produces a brief electrical seizure in the brain, but because the patient is paralyzed, there is no movement in the body. No muscle spasms, no jerky movements, and the patient wakes up several minutes later not recalling the process. It is an experience very similar to having a minor surgical procedure such as having wisdom teeth pulled. The seizures are usually provoked by a shock on only one side of the brain, making the period of memory loss afterwards much less. Unfortunately, the patients still require several seizures to produce a benefit, and there may still be side effects.

Patients who are referred for ECT will typically be scheduled for twelve seizures. Generally, a single seizure is given two to three times a week. Patients usually begin to improve motor function after the fifth or sixth seizure. Depression will start to improve by about the eighth seizure. The side effects are usually minor, consisting primarily of mild memory loss or confusion for a few minutes to a couple of days after each seizure. Sometimes, particularly in the older patient with memory loss or cognitive dysfunction, the postseizure confusion is more likely to be longer and may sometimes prevent the course of treatment from being completed.

The procedure is called ECT because an electric shock is applied to produce a convulsive seizure. A convulsive seizure is one in which there are major muscle contractions, either severe stiffening of the muscles or major muscle jerking, or both. There are other types of seizures, which mostly affect behavior, with little muscle activity. The psychiatric benefit appears to require the type of seizure that involves the whole brain and the muscles. In our modern treatment we paralyze the muscles, but we get the same effect, because it is based on how the brain is affected. Since there are no accepted theories on how ECT makes some psychiatric problems better, there is no explanation as to why eight to twelve seizures are required. In fact, we generally think of seizures as being bad for the brain since seizures disrupt normal electrical activity. How a series of seizures given a few days apart makes the brain work better is another mystery.

In the general population ECT is used primarily to treat severe depression in patients who have not responded to medications. The usual scenario is the patient who has failed three or four antidepressants, is severely depressed, and needs to be treated. ECT is instituted and is usually very helpful. The patient is then usually treated again with antidepressant medications, which, after successful ECT, are usually helpful in keeping the depression under control. In occasional cases, where the medications are still not entirely helpful after the ECT, more seizures may be induced, but at a much lower rate, generally one treatment every three to six weeks instead of two or three each week.

Although I believe that ECT is underutilized in Parkinson's disease (PD) patients, I should point out that it is not a panacea. It does not treat everything, and it isn't always so well tolerated. Even patients who have improved significantly on ECT sometimes refuse to have further treatments, saying only that they don't like it. In non-PD cases, occasional ECT-treated patients will report long-term memory problems, although many studies have been unable to document any long-term memory or cognitive changes after ECT. A major roadblock to ECT in PD patients is dementia. Patients who have memory and thinking problems are much more likely to have a delirium, or confusional state, that may last for a few days after each ECT treatment. This may make it impossible to use, an example of the "cure" being worse than the disease. Some heart ailments, particularly arrhythmias, may make ECT unsafe.

One of the often-unappreciated benefits of ECT is improved motor function. I have seen this in several cases, and it has been the subject of many publications. The explanation for the motor benefit is as mysterious as the benefit for depression. I am not aware that single epileptic seizures in PD patients who also suffer from epilepsy have improved their parkinsonism, yet the controlled, multiple seizures do help PD patients with their mobility. Interestingly the motor improvement usually occurs after four or five ECT treatments, which is generally before the improvement in behavior, which usually begins after a few more seizures. The improvement in mobility after ECT treatment has been so dramatic in some circumstances that some psychiatrists who are highly focused on ECT have recommended using ECT, at least in experimental trials, to treat motor problems in PD patients who have been having difficulty with their medication. I do not think this has ever been done, or at least reported, and I am certain that it is unlikely that any PD specialist would recommend this approach. An important point to keep in mind is that the motor benefits of the ECT are transient, lasting from a few days to a few weeks, but never more than that.

In occasional cases, where ECT has been successful and medications have not been very helpful, even after a course of ECT treatments, the ECT is given in an ongoing manner. This is called "maintenance ECT," which means that the ECT is given once every few weeks, usually in addition to medications. It is not clear whether the maintenance ECT provides the same benefit in motor function as the initial series of ECT treatments. I have followed a few patients who have had maintenance ECT and have not seen significant motor improvements continue, and certainly when they do occur, the benefit is much less.

When should a PD patient be considered for ECT? I think that severe depression is clearly one reason for using ECT if medications have not been successful or the depression is so severe that it is thought that waiting four to six weeks to see if the chosen drug regimen will work, possibly taking several more weeks to then increase the dose or change drug regimens, is intolerable. Since ECT usually begins to help depression after about six to eight seizures, this may mean two to three weeks, obviously a much shorter period of time. There have been reports of ECT improving psychotic symptoms such as hallucinations and delusions that did not respond to antipsychotic drugs and severe anxiety that was unresponsive to the usual medications for that. These are not "recognized" indications for ECT, that is, most psychiatrists would not recommend ECT to treat severe anxiety or psychosis. The number of reports in the literature are very few, and they are case reports or very small series, not truly scientific studies. However, after assessments by psychiatric colleagues, I've referred some patients with truly intractable delusions, present for several years and unresponsive to antipsychotic medications, and patients with devastating anxiety, who have done extremely well.

The problem of anxiety, in particular, is one that I believe has been underestimated. In part this may be due to how we classify psychiatric disorders. Anxiety is often associated with depression, so that doctors focus on the depression as the underlying diagnosis, and some patients have a syndrome called "agitated depression," in which patients are overly active both in thought and action while being severely depressed. Since most patients I've seen who are so severely anxious that they need to be hospitalized are also depressed to some extent, one can often "justify" the use of ECT to treat severe anxiety.

This chapter certainly doesn't mean to imply that all patients with these problems should be offered ECT. I do think, however, that it should be considered when all else fails and that many neurologists oppose ECT without having any experience.

Patients having ECT may be able to receive it as outpatients or may need to be in the hospital. Maintenance ECT is almost always given to outpatients.

17

. . . .

Misperception

The behavioral topics I addressed earlier in the book are different in nature than the topics addressed here. The other chapters focus on emotionally based issues, whereas this chapter is aimed at describing some of the ways in which Parkinson's disease (PD) patients, as the result of their disorder, may see the world differently than the rest of us in a "real-world" fashion.

PD patients often have abnormalities in visual–spatial perception. A common and very concrete issue to consider is the patient who sits down when not properly aligned with the chair. Luckily this doesn't happen to most people, but once present it is a consistent problem that is very difficult to overcome, and I doubt that one can be trained out of it. Typically such patients will attempt to sit in a chair when they are still several inches away from it, and often when they are at an angle so that one leg is close to the chair and the other is a fair distance away. So, when they sit, they end up partly, but not completely, on the chair. In the worst-case scenarios they have too little of their rear end on the chair and they fall to the ground. No matter how many times they are reminded, they can't seem to get it right. And there is a reason for this. PD alters how they see the world. I view the difference as being analogous to seeing an object at the bottom of a stream or a fish tank. The object looks like it's in one place, but if you push a straight object at it you discover that the water has altered your line of sight. Similar problems occur in PD, hence the chair problem. Luckily, if the patient can be educated to touch the armrests before sitting, that overrides the visual image and the patient is almost always able to sit without a problem.

A closely related problem may occur with driving. Family members will accompany a patient to the office and when I ask about driving, the patient will say there's no problem but the spouse may report that the patient always is on one side of the lane, and never stays in the middle. Furthermore, when this is discussed while driving, the patient will argue and insist that he is in the middle of the lane. Similarly, the PD patient may see a car coming as he's trying to make a turn, but misjudge the distance between the cars, or the speed of the oncoming car.

One of the tests we often put new patients through is the "clock drawing test," in which we draw a circle and ask the patient to fill in the numbers. In the "classic" PD clock, the numbers are drawn correctly, although smaller than usual, but they fill up a much smaller circle than the circle drawn by the doctor, leaving a large halo around the drawn numbers. The patient perceives the clock face as normal, whereas all others wonder why the numbers are all cramped in a circle near the top.

A second, related misperception is bodily orientation in space. While we may think of the PD patient who falls backwards when standing up, who puts his feet in front of his center of gravity when getting up from a chair, who can't manipulate his body in the bed in order to turn over, as having motor problems, that is, problems with muscle movement, the real problem lies in a loss of knowing where one's center of gravity is. For example, some patients with severe PD, who cannot get up from a chair without being pulled, will resist the pull, even though they want to get up. Once upright, they may still be leaning backwards, but when asked where they would fall if they let go, they will often think they would fall forward when, in fact, they would fall backward. Interestingly, after they are upright and are properly balanced, they will not fall forward or backward and seem to regain an overall sense of balance. Similarly, some patients, when asked to stand up, will put their feet in front of the chair, and in front of their center of gravity, so that when they attempt to stand, they go backward or don't move at all. They lack the innate sensation of where they must plant their feet in order to move their center of gravity in order to stand up. It would be like hitting a cue ball in billiards off center.

A third related issue is the lack of concern of the patient who is severely tilted to one side. Some PD patients will tilt dramatically to one side and be content, staying endlessly in a posture, almost parallel to the ground, while seated in a chair, one arm and half the trunk over the armrest. They do not complain of pain or discomfort, and do not seek to be righted. I believe this may partly be due to motor dysfunction but is primarily due to a problem with the brain sensing up and down.

The fourth related problem is the difficulty turning in bed or getting up from the floor after a fall. The brain simply can't coordinate the movements that take advantage of leverage, knowing where the center of gravity is, and applying it to advantage. PD patients tend to be like turtles on their back, unable to grasp a purchase on something that will allow them to turn or to stand.

A nonvisual spatial problem of abnormal perception involves dyskinesias. These are squirmy or jerky movements that are always due to PD medications, and usually due to an oversensitivity that develops over years of medication use. One of the peculiar aspects of this syndrome is that patients routinely underestimate the severity of the movements. When mild, they don't perceive them as being present. When moderate they are felt to be mild and when severe they are experienced as moderate. Only the very severe movements tend to bother the patient. It turns out that this under-appreciation is common to all disorders in which people experience these dyskinetic movements. And they do occur in several other conditions. What is even more interesting was the result of a study, unfortunately based only on a single patient, in which the patient was asked to rate the severity of her movements. She was then asked to look at herself in the mirror and rate them again. And finally, she was shown a video-tape of herself that was made as she was rating herself by looking in the mirror. The patient's rating of herself was the same when look-ing in the mirror and when not looking in the mirror, but she found it much more severe when she saw herself on the video. The hypoth-esized explanation is that when she looked in the mirror, seeing herself in "real time" her brain was "expecting" the movements, but when she watched the video, the movements were out of phase with the movements she had, which allowed her to perceive them more accurately. This was considered a "feed forward" problem, mean-ing that the process in the brain that created the movements was sending messages to the brain to expect the movements as "normal" and therefore not consider them as out of the ordinary. This would explain why she didn't perceive them by herself, or when looking in the mirror, but did perceive them when they were "out of synch" on the video.

Another nonvisual misperception is weakness. Many people with PD feel weak, particularly in their legs. They often report that their legs feel as if they're made of lead or concrete. On testing, the legs have normal strength, but patients who cannot control the coor-dination properly often feel this problem as a weakness. Oftentimes PD patient will report feeling weak all over, which usually means that their PD medications aren't working. James Parkinson called the dis-ease "the shaking palsy," meaning tremor and weakness. He believed that PD patients did, in fact, have muscular weakness. Some famous neurologists believed this as well, but we no longer think this is true, although PD patients will have difficulty with repeated activities, so that their muscles do fatigue earlier. In a study on my own patients, about 40% reported feeling an abnormal sense of weakness.

While the frequent problem of speech alteration has been well known for a long time, it is not well understood. There are several different types of speech problems that may occur, including stuttering, poor articulation, overly rapid speech, and reduced volume. Patients are always aware of the stuttering, and generally of the poor articulation, but often not of the reduced volume. Many patients believe they are talking at a normal or even a loud volume, when, in fact, their speech is soft and difficult for others to understand. This is particularly common on the telephone, but also occurs in face-to-face interactions. Patients can overcome this by consciously talking louder than they think they should.

A very serious problem that I've uncovered is the patient who falls very frequently. We did a study to determine how often PD patients fell in the three months since I had seen them last. Most patients didn't fall at all, but a substantial fraction did suffer one or more falls. We scored how many times each patient had fallen, and the number didn't vary too much. Most fell only once or twice, some fell more, sometimes as much as once each week, but we had a few outliers who fell every day, or sometimes even more than that. I wondered how this could happen. What could be a greater learning experience than falling down? The first explanation, that the patients were demented and simply didn't recall that they had a walking or balance problem, was clearly not the answer. These patients could tell me how they fell. They remembered the falls and knew that they fell frequently, so the explanation was not so simple.

The real explanation, I believe, based on what patients told me, is that although they knew that they were at high risk of falling, they felt confident that they wouldn't fall *this* time. They felt strong. They felt that their balance was okay at the moment. Of course, having fallen so many times without major injury, they were less fearful of falling than a lot of other patients, but the real issue was poor insight. They simply didn't stop and think. They were impulsive. This is a form of disinhibition, a problem in which people stop considering the consequences of their actions and act without thinking. It is generally an uncommon problem in PD, but does occur in the impulse control disorders discussed in Chapter 11, where the problem is related to PD medication.

I have not figured out how to solve this problem. After all, if a fall doesn't teach you a lesson, what will? I try to teach patients that every fall is unexpected. If it was expected, it wouldn't happen. If something only occurs when unexpected, the only way to reduce the risk is to assume it may happen at any moment. Unfortunately, reason is not very helpful in altering behavior, and even though my explanation may be somewhat useful for the caregiver, it nevertheless doesn't make life any easier when the patient falls again later that day, thinking he didn't need the cane or walker. After all, it was only a few steps to the bathroom.

18

· ·

Placebo

One of the least well-understood responses to treatment is the response to placebo. A placebo is a treatment that is believed to be inert, that is, to have no physiological action. Placebo pills are often called "sugar pills" or "dummy" medications. Placebos are very important because they are at the heart of modern experimental therapeutics. Almost all treatments, and certainly all medications, that have been developed in the last 50 years or so have tested against placebo to prove that they are both effective and safe. The reason for this lies in the issue of "mind over matter," or "the power of positive thinking."

Placebos aren't necessarily medications. Sometimes placebos are other "sham" treatments, such as "make believe" surgery or other "make believe" procedures. The effect of a placebo can be thought of as being similar to hypnosis. A hypnotized person may believe that something sour is sweet, or that a painful injection is not painful and perhaps even ticklish. I've seen hypnotized doctors believe that they had lost their navel (belly button) and ask for help finding it. One study looked at the effect of a "sham" spinal tap (lumbar puncture) on walking ability in people with a rare neurological condition that is supposed to improve after a spinal tap. Half the group got the numbing injection and the spinal tap, and half only got the numbing medicine. Neither could tell if they had had the spinal tap because the numbing medicine prevented their feeling the needle. Both groups had remarkable improvement. There was no difference between the two groups, so the researchers had to conclude that spinal taps didn't help the patients' walking any more than the simple expectation of improvement helped.

It is very common, almost the rule, that placebos are very helpful in treatment trials. This means that an experimental medication, even if not medically helpful, may nevertheless show positive results as a result of the placebo effect. This is the reason that the Food and Drug Administration almost always requires that a new treatment be tested against placebo. Helping a condition is not enough. A study needs to prove that the treatment helps significantly more than the placebo. Thus, we have the concept of a "placebo-controlled" trial (a "trial" is often called a "study," so the two words are used interchangeably). A "control" is a comparison subject. In a controlled trial, each person with PD who is given the active treatment is matched with a Parkinson's disease (PD) patient who receives the placebo. Neither the doctor nor the participants know whether they are getting one or the other until the study is over, keeping everyone "honest," that is, from influencing the outcome by reporting more side effects or benefits, or both, if they find out they're on the active treatment, or fewer benefits or side effects if they find out they're on the placebo.

There have been many research studies in which an experimental medication has been used in a placebo-controlled trial and been found not to work, meaning it didn't do better than the placebo, or was harmful. If a drug company is testing a medication and finds out it isn't helpful, they stop testing, to avoid wasting more money. On rare occasions, patients who were in a trial and found the treatment helpful have threatened to sue the drug company after a trial had been completed, to make the company continue giving them the drug. In some instances these patients were found to have been taking the placebo.

There have been many studies of the "placebo response." Some studies have shown that a certain colored pill produced a greater response than pills in other colors, or that pills might produce a better response than capsules. Very often the demeanor of the research team may make a treatment more or less effective. If the team acts as if the treatment is sure to work, then the subject is much more likely to report a benefit than if the team seems very pessimistic. Some of the older readers of this may remember Chairman Mao's Little Red Book, widely distributed in communist China in the 1960s. The book was a collection of quotes from the leader of the country and was said to possess magical powers. Those who believed in it were able to have operations without anesthesia because of their belief in the power of the book.

There are two important studies to discuss here. One has to do with pain. Pain perception is very clearly related to the person's psyche. We know that in emergencies people may not feel any pain, which in other circumstances would be intolerable. A soldier with a severe injury may keep fighting and acting as if not injured, whereas the same person may complain about the pain from a small blister. Pain is blunted by the body's own endorphins, hormones that respond to pain perception. In a study in which research subjects whose pain had improved with placebo were given naloxone, a drug that blocks the effects of opiate pain medications and endorphins, the placebo stopped working. This implies that the body somehow translates the mind's belief in the power of the placebo to actually increase the body's endorphins to suppress the pain.

In spectacular experiments in PD, patients were told what the chances were that they would receive a pill with L-Dopa versus a placebo pill. As the percentage chance of the active drug increased, the likelihood of responding to placebo increased as well. Thus the anticipation of a response produced the response. More impressive, however, was another experiment, in which the amount of dopamine released was measured in PD patients. Dopamine is, of course, in the brain, not in the blood, so the amount of dopamine was measured using a positron emission tomography (PET) scan. When patients were given

L-Dopa and their motor function improved, the PET scan showed that the amount of dopamine in the brain had also increased. They then measured the amount of dopamine released when patients were given the placebo. In the patients who had a placebo response—that is, their movements improved on placebo—they found an increase in dopamine that was similar to the level that occurred in the PD patients who actually received L-Dopa. The placebo-treated patients who did not respond to the placebo showed no increase in dopamine. Thus, the mind was able to "trick" the brain into making more dopamine to improve movement.

How this process works remains a mystery. Obviously, if we could harness the placebo response, we'd be able to have patients treat themselves without drugs for a number of conditions. There is a definite and clearly demonstrated power to "positive thinking." People with a "positive" attitude with cancer live longer and have fewer medication side effects. The placebo response may be similar to that. We don't know.

The placebo effect does, however, underscore the importance of the psyche in PD. We know from the time of James Parkinson, that mental attitude has important effects in PD. Patients with tremor always report that it gets worse with anxiety, stress, and excitement. We know that some patients can't walk well when others are looking at them, although they can walk well when alone. Patients who are barely able to walk become transformed when they go on vacation to another location. The placebo response is closely related to all these types of psychic responses to the environment.

And we should not forget that there is an opposite to the placebo response, often called the "nocebo" response. The "nocebo" response is a negative response to an inert intervention. For example, just as people may improve with a placebo, many patients will report getting worse, or having side effects. When drug studies report the side effects of an experimental drug, it is always compared to the side effects of the placebo, since headache, nausea, dizziness, constipation, and a variety of other problems seem to occur with anything (or nothing).

APPENDIX A

· ·

Winning the Battle but Losing the War: Many Silver Linings Are in Clouds

A patient with Parkinson's disease (PD) has been suffering for years. Despite the best possible care, both in his doctor's office and at home, he declines, becomes increasingly dependent, and, perhaps worst of all, fluctuates so much and so randomly during the day that he may feel strong enough to go out shopping alone at one point but then get "frozen" in place at the store and require rescue to bring him home by ambulance. This patient, mentally intact, is referred for deep brain stimulation (DBS) surgery. He is tested in the standard fashion, which includes a very complete medical history, review of all PD drug regimens to see if other approaches may be tried, an evaluation with the patient off medication, an evaluation with the patient on medication, a neuropsychological examination, and a psychiatric examination, all before meeting with the neurosurgeon to review the procedure and the potential adverse consequences.

He goes through the procedure and is dramatically improved. His family reports that the day of the surgery is the date of his "rebirth." That day marks the beginning of his new life, a miraculous transformation from his presurgical bondage to his disease.

This is the stuff that doctors' dreams are made of (especially surgeons)! How god-like we are (sometimes)!

Unfortunately, six months later things don't look so good. His Parkinson's is extremely well controlled. He doesn't fluctuate anymore. He is always "on." He drives, has resumed playing golf, and is well enough to go back to work. The patient is separated from his wife and children and is still not employed. He's depressed. His initial enthusiasm has vanished. As they say in the trade, "The surgery was a success but the patient died." It is a sad and fascinating phenomenon that was brought to my attention only recently. Some patients, with sudden and dramatic improvements in health may actually decompensate psychosocially. This happens in PD. It happens with epilepsy surgery as well. And, I'll bet it happens with other dramatically transforming interventions too.

With the loss of disability and dependency, a number of things may happen. When positive, the shackles are broken, the caregiver is freed, the patient returns to work or other gainful activities, the old family pattern is restored, and everyone rejoices. When negative, the caregiver loses her role in life. No longer the suffering martyr, she now has to go back to work, spend more time with the extended family, and pay more attention to things less rewarding. The patient no longer has a slave-on-call. He no longer can say, "My PD is bad, please do this...." Suddenly there are responsibilities that haven't been there for years. Suddenly there is no longer a reason to justify special entitlements. Having to take an active and major role in family dynamics in place of a major but passive role may be unwelcome. Maybe the family no longer centers around the sick person anymore. The spotlight is off.

This has been described in epilepsy surgery as well. When patients are chosen carefully for epilepsy surgery, even those with daily, debilitating seizures may become seizure-free. In fact, about 75% do. Patients who may have had one or more spells daily, suffering from the terrible effects of the seizures plus the prolonged and sometimes equally disabling postictal states, become normal. Not only do the seizures and the postictal states stop, but the medication use goes down, along with their side effects of sleepiness, fatigue, mental dullness, incoordination, decreased interest, and so on. With excellent seizure results coupled with a lack of neurological adverse effects, the benefits of epilepsy surgery are as dramatic as those in well-chosen PD patients. Yet in one recent study, successful surgical outcomes were associated with a 2% suicide rate, a 5% depression rate, a 35% rate of "restructuring family dynamics," and a 12% grief reaction "over lost years."

When I think about these observations I conclude that while these outcomes are understandable, maybe even predictable to some of us, they certainly are a surprise to me. I do not reflect on these outcomes and say, "Gee, we should have thought of that. Of course family dynamics will change and those results are always unpredictable." I can't imagine myself or any of my colleagues sitting down to initiate our program in deep brain stimulation surgery in PD saying, "What are we going to do if these people get better?" After all, the whole point of the surgery is to make dramatic improvements. If we don't achieve this we shouldn't be offering it to our patients. We have learned, however, that we must discuss this issue with the patient, the caregiver, and the family, but it's not clear to me what any of us can do with that information. Can anyone refuse a surgical candidate whose parkinsonism we think will benefit from DBS surgery because we're afraid the support system will collapse, or the relationship with the spouse will implode, or something equally dire will occur? I think not, but we can recommend counseling and review the possible negative outcomes of a positive surgical result.

I haven't heard yet of anyone turning off their stimulator to become disabled, but I won't be surprised when it happens.

APPENDIX B

· ·

Chemical Imbalance or Moral Weakness? Personal Responsibility in a Time of Brain Science

William Bennett, Secretary of Education in the Bush senior administration, wrote a best-selling book on morals. It was therefore of great public interest when he was outed as a pathological gambler. Of course, people who make a public point of educating the rest of us on ethics are like the people who lecture us on sexual issues. They are often people trapped by their fears and failings, part fox, part hen, wanting to guard your chicken coops (not theirs).

How much of behavior is "teachable?" Obviously we think that most is or we wouldn't be spending so much time teaching it. We also know that behavior is a brain process and that much depends on the various connections and proportions of the neurotransmitter "humors." The brain is, in simple terms, an organ ("my second most favorite organ," according to Woody Allen) that works along scientific principles, analogous to the "lesser" organs. Of course, these are far more complex and include the most difficult to understand concept, self-knowledge.

Brain alterations cause behavioral changes. Damage the frontal lobes and the ability to experience emotion is blunted or destroyed (frontal lobotomies). Stimulate one tiny region and you may create depression or mania, or cure severe obsessions. Brain diseases cause a variety of dysfunctions as do many medications that act on the brain. Crimes committed during active brain malfunctions are almost always considered the responsibility of the patient and not the disease. "Not guilty by reason of insanity" virtually never results in acquittal, except on television. A schizophrenic who kills someone while in the grip of a delusion is usually punished. Alcohol or drug intoxication does not exculpate responsibility.

Subtle personality alterations, however, are harder to address.

Only after about 25 years of experience using dopamine agonist medications (bromocriptine, pergolide, pramipexole, ropinerole, rotigotine, and lisuride) in Parkinson's disease (PD) did anyone notice that they may cause pathological gambling in people who had never been so inclined. When the medication is lowered the behavior resolves. The patients, being unaware that this is a potential medication effect, notice that they've become interested in this activity that had never interested them before. They do not experience this as a foreign or alien feeling. They are not intoxicated. They are not delirious. Their personality, memory, problem-solving abilities are all intact. It is perhaps analogous to someone deciding that they would like to pursue a new hobby, repairing old cars, starting to knit, becoming a water colorist, and so on. In fact, it is possible that some people on these medications may have begun doing these very things, since the drugs have induced rare cases of severe senseless repetitive behavior disorders. An article in a neurology journal described a PD patient who had, indeed, developed a "calling" to oil painting. The authors thought that this medication was to "blame," but who knows if the patient may have developed such a calling even if she hadn't been on the medications, or developed PD, since they didn't stop the medication to determine if this was a medicine-related behavior?

If the PD patient lost his house at a casino, could he sue the drug company that made the drug for not having this information in the package insert? Could he sue me for not preparing him for this outcome? How much is the drug's fault, and how much is the patient's? Who's responsible? If the drug is responsible, then isn't it possible that compulsive gamblers not on these medications may simply have genetic abnormalities causing similar chemical imbalances that mimic this process? And if this is true, does it imply that the courts should be more lenient with them when they declare bankruptcy?

The question here, of course, is where does personal responsibility end and relentless physiology begin? Are the PD patients who developed a desire to gamble different, in some way from other PD patients taking equal amounts of drug; different in some tangible, physiological way? Do they metabolize the drug differently, or do they simply have a "weaker" id, a lesser ability to ward off impulses? Are they morally weaker than the others or do the others simply not have these impulses at all? They do not experience the urge to gamble as foreign. They experience the desire and the pleasure as new, but not alien. The PD patients who don't gamble usually chuckle when asked about gambling, and report that they have not felt any urge to buy scratch tickets, or go to the gambling tables. They've had no impulse to resist.

A doctor with PD acts inappropriately with a patient of the opposite sex. He loses his license. Is it a medication-related problem? Can he practice again if his PD medications are altered? Who's to blame? How do you detect a problem that does not seem out of place? How do we decide if a behavioral change is part of a disease process, due to the treatment, or simply intrinsic to the person's personality? Most people who gamble, pathologically or not, do not have PD. None of them take the offending drug. There are many paths to the same outcome.

I believe that people should be held responsible for their actions. I also believe, however, that there are different levels of responsibility, so that the existence of certain brain disorders should mitigate punishment. A postseizure patient who, in a confused state, hurts a bystander trying to help him, is not responsible for his actions, at least not if he's been taking his medications. A patient who acts out dream-behavior and does something bad while asleep can't be deemed responsible, unless he had refused treatment for this problem. But with these very rare exceptions, most others are indeed responsible for their actions. Sometimes that responsibility is shared with the doctor providing the medicine.

Most of the time no one knows how irrational, pathological, or "alien" behaviors originate. The fact that some of these can be induced by medications that appear to produce exquisitely isolated behaviors, such as gambling, but not other impulsive or compulsive behaviors, suggests that our personalities and habits may be governed more by a multitude of rather simple chemical relationships than by years of ethical teaching. Of course, the education may produce the harmonious chemical balance underlying the state of appropriate grace, but a mild perturbation of one neurotransmitter in an enormously complex soup may put the whole system out of balance.

It is a true observation, but daunting, for it undermines our confidence in the very notion of personal responsibility.

There is no data to indicate whether sanctimonious hypocrisy may also be the result of a simple chemical problem.

APPENDIX C

· ·

Urban Myth: L-Dopa Stops Working in Five Years

I can't explain why I didn't write this article sooner, or why someone else didn't write it or popularize it long ago. I have heard concerns both from patients and from health professionals, even including an occasional neurologist, that L-Dopa stops working in five years. This notion, if true, should generate a lot of concern about even starting the drug, since who would like to know that in five years they were going to fall off a cliff?

Let me start by reviewing how L-Dopa works. The major problem (unfortunately not the only problem) in Parkinson's disease (PD) is that the brain cells that make dopamine (chemical shorthand for di-ortho-phenylalanine) are attacked, weaken and die. Almost all our treatments for PD focus on trying to restore a more normal chemical balance in the brain, with a dopamine deficiency being the central problem. L-Dopa is our most important medication in treating PD. Interestingly it is not actually the active ingredient in helping PD patients. L-Dopa first gets into the bloodstream and is then taken up by the brain cells that make dopamine. These cells then convert L-Dopa to dopamine and thereby make more of it, enabling the brain to function more normally. In our model of how the brain works, we can think of these brain cells as being tiny chemical factories which make dopamine. The amount of dopamine each brain cell makes depends on how much L-Dopa it has to work with, so that the more L-Dopa available, up to a point, the more dopamine gets produced.

This means that as long as there are brain cells still alive that make dopamine, L-Dopa will continue to work. This also means that as the number of these cells decline, the less of an impact the L-Dopa is going to make. If you imagine having 1,000 factories making dopamine at maximum capacity at one time, and several years later having 500 factories, you can see that less dopamine is going to be produced, so that the drug will have a reduced effect. However, it is extremely rare for PD patients to get to a point where they have so few dopamine-producing brain cells left that the drug has no effect.

So where did the myth arise that L-Dopa "stops working in five years?" I think that some people got confused by a very important observation that many PD patients taking L-Dopa develop side effects from being on the medication for a long time and that half the patients will have some sort of side effect within five years. These "long-term" side effects are different than the "short-term" side effects. Short-term side effects, like sleepiness or nausea or realistic dreams, usually develop as soon as the medication is started, whereas long-term side effects typically develop after a patient has been taking the medication for years. The short-term side effects, if they occur, usually go away within a few weeks.

The most common long-term side effects of L-Dopa are dyskinesias and fluctuating responses. Dyskinesia is a technical term composed of "dys," which means abnormal, and "kinesia," which means movement. A dyskinesia is an abnormal movement. PD patients who have taken L-Dopa for years often develop involuntary movements that look like "the fidgets," or like stretching movements. Patients often describe them as "swaying" if they occur while standing, or "dancing," but may also be "squirming." They are not usually bothersome to the patient and generally are more noticed by the family than the patient.

These movements are directly related to the amount of PD medications taken and will go away when the medications are reduced.

The second long-term problem is that of fluctuations. When this first occurs, the doses of the L-Dopa, "wear off," which means that it doesn't last as long as it used to, so the benefit begins to decline before the next dose is taken. With time, the response to each dose sometime varies so that one dose lasts for four hours while another lasts for only two hours, or something along that line. Occasionally a patient will report that some doses do not produce any benefit at all. This probably has to do with problems absorbing the medication, and certainly does not mean the pills are defective.

I believe that L-Dopa always is helpful as long as there are enough dopamine-producing cells in the brain, and it is a rare patient who has so few cells left that a dose of L-Dopa produces no improvement in movement. After five years many patients have problems with their L-Dopa, but they all have some benefit. It is an error to postpone taking L-Dopa due to fear that it will stop working in five years.

APPENDIX D

· ·

Staging Parkinson's Disease

I am often asked by patients what stage of Parkinson's disease (PD) that they are in. I then explain the following, as to why that is not an important issue.

Staging most disease is important in predicting how long people will live or how well they can function. This is particularly important in cancer and heart disease. Different cancers have different systems for staging as experience has accumulated to distinguish how ominous it is to have cancer spread to local lymph nodes, or distant nodes, above the diaphragm, or below the diaphragm, in the bone marrow or not, and so on. So Stage 2b in one disease may have a very different prognosis than Stage 2b in another form of cancer, but each will be associated with a certain chance of surviving for a specified period.

This is not true for staging in PD. The staging system we use is based on a famous paper written by Margaret Hoehn and Melvin Yahr in 1967. Their paper was the first large study of the effect of L-Dopa on disease progression. In order to assess how the disease progressed, they had to develop a system to rate the severity. It wouldn't do, for example, to say "mild," "moderate," and "severe," as the readers would want to know what they meant by these terms. And, as I'll make clear below, this is still the problem that has kept neurologists from developing a better system.

In the Hoehn–Yahr (HY) staging system, stage 1.0 means that the PD is limited to one side of the body. Tremor, rigidity, reduced arm swing, slowness are present only on one side. Stage 2.0 refers to problems affecting both sides, although one side may be only minimally involved. I should state that there are experts who think there is no such thing as stage 1.0, that everyone with involvement on one side has some deficit on the other, but that it might be hard to see because there isn't a normal side to compare with and also because we know from autopsy evidence that PD always affects both sides.

In the original HY system, there were no stages 1.5 and 2.5. These were added later as refinements. In stage 1.5 only one side is affected but one can see symmetric problems on both sides such as reduced facial expression, stooped posture, or reduced arm swing. In stage 2.5 both sides are involved plus there is a mild impairment of balance but not loss of balance. To test for this the patient is told that he will be pulled backwards and to take a step back to try to prevent a fall. The patient is then pulled backwards firmly. It is considered normal to take one or two steps but if three or more steps are taken and balance is recovered, it is considered stage 2.5 (or 1.5 if there are no signs of PD on the better side).

Stage 3 refers to PD with impaired balance, defined by loss of balance when pulled backwards so that the examiner must catch the patient to prevent a fall. Stage 4 is defined differently in different places. In some places it is defined by the need for an assistive device or a person to help a patient walk, whereas in others it refers to severe impairment but where some walking is possible. Stage 5 means unable to walk.

The first problem with the HY staging is that it is based purely on mobility and takes no account of mental, behavior, or other non-motor problems. Since every study on health-related quality of life demonstrates that the most important determinants of quality of life in PD patients are nonmotor behavioral problems such as dementia, depression, fatigue, and sleep disorders, it may be irrelevant if the motor symptoms are mild but the patient is depressed and demented. His disease has severely altered his life, yet he may have stage 1.0, seemingly mild disease.

The second problem has to do with the impact of the motor symptoms. A person may have stage 1.0, the lowest possible stage, with a small amount of tremor, a little slowness and reduced arm swing, but look and work normally; or the PD may be very severe on the one side so that one arm is almost useless but the other side is normal. If the affected side is nondominant, for example, the left side is affected in a right-handed person, the disease is annoying but may not interfere with work. The same stage, 1.0, affecting the right side may be completely debilitating. Yet they are both stage 1.0.

Unlike staging for cancer, higher stages may be less severe than lower stages. For example, a person who has minimal motor dysfunction but has it on both sides, has stage 2.0, which might be far less severe than someone who has severe motor problems on only the dominant side. Similarly, someone with stage 3, meaning there is a balance problem, may have very mild motor dysfunction and have less impairment than someone with stage 1.0.

One can easily imagine many scenarios where a lower stage is associated with more severe disease than a higher stage. And even if we look at scoring systems such as the unified Parkinson's disease rating scale, in which there is a point score for tremor, rigidity, speech, slowness, and so on, one sees the same confounding problems. For example, we rate tremor in each limb, and chin, from 0, meaning not present, to 4, meaning severe, and similarly for speech. Imagine someone who scores a 5 due to a very minimal tremor in each arm, leg, and chin. Compare this to a person with no tremor but speech that is totally incomprehensible, which would rate a 4. Thus, without seeing the actual patient, one would be misled to think that the person with a 5 was worse than the one with a 4, where the opposite is the case.

Severity of PD is currently not really measurable. We currently rate different aspects of PD differently and often use multiple different scales. It affects people in so many different ways that it defies methods for comparison, just as it has been impossible so far to measure what we mean when we say disease progression. We have good methods for measuring the motor symptoms of PD. We add points for tremor, stiffness, slowness, posture, walking, and so on and come up with a number, and that is how we currently test new treatments for PD. Does the treatment reduce that number? Does it slow the worsening of that number? We also have methods for rating the nonmotor symptoms, such as pain, fatigue, sleepiness, and methods for rating the impact of the motor symptoms, such as drooling, penmanship, and speech, but there is no single score than can capture the real impact of the disease. How should one compare someone whose speech is unintelligible but is able to do almost anything else, to someone who can communicate clearly but has severe tremors and needs a walker?

The HY scale is useful for looking at populations of PD patients but is not useful for assessing a single person. It helps us understand how various treatments alter the progression of motor problems in large groups. The severity of your own PD is really a matter of how severely it affects your life. A number can never capture this.

APPENDIX E

. . . .

There's Only One Reason to Nag

Some of the lessons that doctors learn are incorporated into clinical practice but may never get written down because these common sense, hard-learned observations aren't "publishable." They comprise the "art" of medical practice.

One of the central problems in Parkinson's disease (PD) is the difficulty in doing two things at the same time. There is a loss of our "automatic pilot," the part of the brain that allows us to do many complex tasks without thinking about them. As one of my patients put it, "my good hand does what it's supposed to do but my Parkinson hand has to be told what to do." This causes a great deal of slowness because the patient has to guide the hand and not think about the next step.

PD patients don't blink as much as normal people, hence the staring expression, and they don't swallow as much as normal people, hence the pooling of saliva, or the drooling. There is a problem with their "set point" for doing these small things that occur unconsciously. It's like having a thermostat that's always a little bit off. Normal people blink a certain number of times per minute, and PD patients blink a bit less. Not a big deal for most, and "easily" remedied. Just ask the PD person to blink more! Unfortunately, or fortunately, most PD patients have better things to think about than blinking or swallowing so that they can't think about blinking or swallowing all day long. It's the same with writing too small. The patient can write larger, but concentrating on writing larger interferes with thinking about what is being written.

Everyone seems to understand this, but a very similar problem occurs with posture and arm swing. PD patients have a stooped posture, and they also often tilt to one side. The spouse often arrives in the room and tells me, "I keep telling him to stand up straight," or, "I keep reminding him to swing his arms." I then respond, "But it never works does it?" "Well, it does for about a minute." And the reason it doesn't last is just like the reason PD patients can't increase their blink or their swallow rate.

For whatever reason, clearly related to their PD, their brain wants something different than is normal. The brain says to blink less, swallow less, write small, talk softly, stoop the shoulders, shuffle, and while each of these problems can be overridden, they can only be overridden consciously—that is, while people are thinking about one particular problem. Unfortunately there are lots of other things to think about, like what's for dinner, why the Red Sox are crashing again, or if the grandson will get into his first-choice college. No one can think about their posture all day, and especially not about their blinking, their swallowing, their speech volume, and smiling, all at the same time.

This applies to arm swing as well. It is rare that PD patients can make their arms swing normally. It is easy to detect PD patients who consciously swing their arms to look normal because it is difficult to synchronize the movements with the rhythm of the stride.

I try to get spouses and friends to understand that telling the patient to stand up straight never accomplishes anything. It is nagging and only is helpful if the patient *wants* to be reminded, perhaps at a social event or for a photograph. Telling the spouse to stop nagging is greatly appreciated by the patient. And the spouse often appreciates this as well. Most people don't like to nag. They do it only because they feel they must, as part of their "job" as caregiver, booster, facilitator, and so on. It is helpful for spouses and caregivers to hear what the limits are. "Should I nag more? After all he's not standing up straight and if I bother him enough maybe he'll straighten out." It helps to be told not to do it. The spouse can tell the children, "No, I'm not going to bug him anymore. The doctor said he can't help it and this is nagging."

A more difficult problem is tilting. Some PD patients tilt to one side like the Leaning Tower of Pisa. Some patients will tilt so much that their head is on the armrest of the chair and their arm is on the floor. The most amazing thing is that the patient is rarely uncomfortable from this. It looks like torture, and I certainly wouldn't want to sit like that, but the patients who do sit with their head almost parallel to the ground are not bothered. It doesn't help to say, "Sit up straight." The brains in these patients are confused about what is straight, and what up and down are. They usually can't do it, and even when they do, it's for a limited amount of time before they tilt back to their starting position. The best thing to do in these cases is to stuff the chair with pillows and try to keep them as erect as possible.

I don't know what to do about nagging people who fall. I have been impressed by how many PD patients fall in particular situations that they know are problematic and should be able to anticipate. Most patients fall when they try to turn and their feet stick to the ground. So, why don't they simply learn to cope with this by stopping, turning with a few small steps, or by leaning against a wall? I've asked some patients this and I always get a shrug. I also hear from the caregiver that the patient is constantly being told, "Be careful. Turn slowly." "Don't take your hands off the walker." Yet it happens daily or more. I used to say the same thing. "Stop and think before you turn."

One day I had a sudden insight. There are not many stronger stimuli for learning than a very bad experience. If you do something that results in a very bad outcome, you avoid doing that thing again. If you stick a fork in the socket you learn with a single experience to never do that again. Why is it that a PD patient who falls can do the same thing over and over again? I don't know, but I realized one day that if a fall won't teach a patient the danger, then my telling them or their spouse's nagging isn't very likely to help either.

What's the solution? I don't know. It's hard to keep from trying to help. On the other hand, we must learn to avoid nagging. Nagging is demoralizing for the nagger and the one being nagged. The nagger feels ignored and the one being nagged feels misunderstood or morally weak, as if not trying hard enough.

Nagging about exercising is good, though. You can always nag each other about exercising more. It's good for everybody.

APPENDIX F

· ·

Why You Should Not Go to the Emergency Department (And Why You Should!)

I am occasionally called by an emergency department (ED) physician to let me know that Mr. Smith is being evaluated for "freezing" or increased tremors or some other aspect of his Parkinson's disease (PD), and I am asked for advice. Usually I advise the ED doctor to tell the patient to call me the next day and get him out of the ED before something bad happens.

The number of times I've heard the same story, "I went to the ED last week because my PD got so bad I couldn't stand it anymore! And what did they do? They kept me waiting six hours, did a chest x-ray, a brain CT scan, a cardiogram, and a bunch of urine and blood tests and sent me home. And you know they didn't know anything about Parkinson's disease! They never heard of dyskinesias or 'off' periods or even some of my drugs."

It's not the ED's fault. It's the patient and families' and perhaps the PD doctors' fault as well. A trip to the ED may be useful for evaluating anything except PD. Never go to the ED because your PD is worse! You should go if you think you have an infection making it worse, or if you have fallen and are worried about a broken bone or a blood clot on the brain, but if you have bad PD problems that you've been working on with your neurologist, and some time when the doctor's unavailable the PD takes a sudden turn for the worse, I will guarantee that you will be lucky to leave the ED with only a few hours wasted and tablespoons of blood lost. ED doctors do not know much about PD. The better ones will tell you this and advise you to call your PD doctor the next day. Sometimes patients are admitted to their local hospital where their PD specialist may not be able to see them. Then someone who meets them once for twenty minutes or so alters everything that took three years to get into place.

Now, I don't mean to imply that one should never go to the ED, but I do mean that you should never go because your PD is worse without talking to your PD doctor first. Let me provide some scenarios because it is sometimes not so straightforward. Basically, PD patients are relatively stable over weeks at a time. By this I mean "good" patients who reliably respond to the medications stay that way, perhaps developing mildly increased scuffing or tremor or dyskinesias. Patients with moderate to severe fluctuations remain fluctuating no matter how we adjust medications. If we're lucky an adjustment will add one good hour and if we're unlucky we may lose an hour. Some days are good, some days are bad. The parameters of these changes are generally well known but change slowly over time. A person with only two good "on" hours per day may panic if there's a day without any "good" time and will experience it as a terrible, excruciatingly bad day. But in the context of the illness it really was only a little worse, 14 hours "off" increased to 16 hours "off." Of course, the patient and family report that "two hours 'on' went to zero," hence a complete loss of function. While this is certainly cause for grief and concern, it's not cause for alarm and all the brain CT scans and blood tests are not going to teach the ED doctors any new tricks your PD doctor doesn't already know and probably has already tried.

When a patient whose PD has been stable suddenly deteriorates, then reasons other than the PD itself must be suspected. Mild pneumonia, bladder infection, and sometimes other, more serious, nonneurologic problems may exacerbate the PD problems. This worsening of the PD is temporary and reverses when the underlying medical problems are treated. The same is true for memory, thinking, and sleepiness. Sudden, persistent declines in concentration and memory usually indicate either an "occult" (hidden) medical problem, such as an infection or thyroid dysfunction, or a medication-related problem.

Too often the ED doctors diagnose "stroke" even when there's nothing to suggest this condition. They hear the words "suddenly got worse" and the only thing ED doctors know that causes sudden worsening is stroke, so the patient gets a CT scan and an unnecessary stay in the hospital. And the hospital is the last place you want to be if you have problems with PD. They screw up your medication schedule, interrupt your sleep, and interfere with your exercise routines.

Problems with the PD? Call your PD doctor. Problems with thinking, memory, concentration, hallucinations, or strange behavior? Call your PD doctor. Needless wastes of time, body fluids, and money, along with potential harm, can be avoided with a call to the doctor who knows your PD best. If your doctor doesn't help you more than the ED doctors, you need a new PD doctor.

Sometimes PD patients *do* develop medical problems that require hospitalization. They may have heart conditions, pneumonia, stroke, or any medical problem that other people get. In addition they may fall and break bones. Some hospitalizations are for elective procedures such as a knee replacement or a rotator cuff repair.

HOSPITALIZATION IS RARELY FOR THE PD ITSELF

Once in the hospital they often run into a series of problems that are so similar, regardless of the hospital or the medical condition, that it is important for the patient and the caregiver to be aware of what is likely to happen and to make proper provisions ahead of time.

First, it is unlikely that PD medications will be given as prescribed by the physician who originally ordered them, unless the nursing staff and attending physician (if he or she is not a neurologist) are explicitly given schedules in advance. If a person takes Sinemet (carbidopa/levodopa) or dopamine agonists, three times a day before meals, the hospital staff frequently transcribes this order into "TID" (an abbreviation for the Latin translation of three times daily), which could result in an 8 a.m., 4 p.m., midnight schedule. A home schedule of 7 a.m., 11 a.m., 3 p.m., 7 p.m. may be translated into a "QID" (four times daily) or "Q6h" (every six hours) schedule of 7 a.m., 1 p.m., 7 p.m., 1 a.m. When the daily schedule gets more complex, with a dopamine agonist at mealtimes, a whole and half tablet of Sinemet scheduled at different times, or when patients take Sinemet on an "as needed" or "demand" schedule (PRN is the hospital term), all hell breaks loose.

Most physicians and nurses are used to dealing with antibiotics, blood pressure, and diabetes medicines where a firm schedule either doesn't matter, or where the aim is to provide a fairly continuous drug level over a 24-hour period. It is not usual hospital policy to allow the patients to take medications when the parients deem necessary or to take their own medications. This requires a physician's approval and most physicians aren't aware that PD patients often take their medicines on a schedule that may seem quite odd to them, but has been developed over years of trial and error.

SUGGESTIONS

1. Be sure that the drug schedule used at home, with time and dose, is understood and copied into the hospital orders (unless whatever changes are made can be explained). Be sure that the Sinemet (carbidopa/levodopa) strength is correct. It comes as 10/100, 25/100, and 25/250 for the standard (immediate release) form, while the long-acting form (Sinemet CR) comes in two strengths, 25/100 and 50/200. The generic formulations of carbidopa/levodopa

and Sinemet have the same colors at the equivalent strengths and can be interchanged.

2. Don't take or give medications on your own. Let the staff know what is supposed to be given and when, including "as needed" doses.

3. Some medication changes can be accepted. Sometimes drugs need to be reduced. Often, simplification of scheduling must be made because the nursing staff cannot deliver drugs exactly on time. Give the staff some leeway.

4. In some cases, patients may be taking medicines not stocked in the hospital pharmacy. This will always be the case when the patient is enrolled in an experimental drug protocol. It is therefore necessary to bring these medicines *in their original bottles*, and the instructions, to the hospital to ensure that doses are not missed.

5. PD patients who fluctuate ("on" and "off" periods) are usually poorly understood in the hospital. The staff frequently think the patient is trying to be "babied" when he turns "off," asking for help in dressing or eating when he had been sauntering down the corridor unassisted only a few minutes earlier. Occasionally dyskinesias, the writhing movements caused by levodopa overmedication or oversensitivity, are thought to be attention-getting tricks rather than involuntary and unwanted movements.

6. The laws governing when medications are given allows about an hour's leeway on either side. Hospital staff are so overworked that it is difficult for the best-intentioned staff to give all the medications on the optimal schedule.

The best provision to solve these problems is an "in-service" teaching session for the nursing staff. Unfortunately, unless there is a knowledgeable nurse or doctor available to do this, this is not done. When this situation does arise, the attending physician should be informed and asked to educate the staff. Oftentimes, giving literature on PD (such as this chapter) to the staff may be very helpful.

You have to keep in mind that the hospital staff wants the patient to be well cared for. When they "blame" the patient, it is usually from ignorance. Always assume that the staff wants what's best for the patient and that they can be taught. Teach them. Explain the situation in a supportive manner, and do not be hostile or take a negative attitude.

I really appreciate your efforts, but I think you may have never taken care of a PD patient with my husband's type of problems before. He is really different than most of the PD patients. Let me explain his situation and give you some literature to read."

"I know you are really understaffed, but it is very important for my husband to get his medications as close to the proper time as possible."

Do not accuse the staff of being incompetent and uncaring. Ask them to call the patient's neurologist.

Confusion is also a major problem for hospitalized patients and particularly older ones. The combined stress of another medical problem superimposed on PD, the changed environment, with strangers invading one's privacy every few minutes, the continuous noise and lights, the degree of helplessness and dependence and the frequent introduction of new drugs often pushes the patient "over the edge" into a delirious state with disorientation, fragmented, and distorted memory, misperceptions of what is going on, and even hallucinations.

This is so common, unfortunately, that it is to be expected. I try to tell my patients and their families before an elective procedure such as a knee replacement or some other operation, that this problem may occur and not to worry. After surgery the confusion is probably due mainly to the effects of anesthesia combined with pain medication and the stress of the surgery itself.

This condition is not caused by a stroke. CT scans, MRIs, EEGs, and various other tests are only rarely indicated. The problem is transient and will disappear once the underlying problem is controlled, physical recovery takes place, and the new medications are stopped.

The best solution for this situation is to comfort the patient and to control the behavior when it threatens her well-being. Physical restraints are sometimes required, but are very disturbing both to the patient and to the family.

Oftentimes physicians use antipsychotic medications such as haloperidol to control abnormal behavior. While haldol may be very useful in most patients, it is to be avoided, if possible, in PD patients because it makes Parkinson's symptoms worse. Quetiapine and clozapine may be used, however, because they do not worsen mobility or stiffness. If an injected drug must be used because the patient won't swallow, then I recommend lorazepam (Ativan) or diazepam (Valium). While it is true that these drugs may worsen the confusion, they generally calm the patient to an extent that behavior problems are less common and less severe. Generally the delirium resolves itself over a few days and the sedative may then be stopped.

If an antipsychotic drug is required, the medication of choice is quetiapine. The second-line drug is clozapine. These are the only antipsychotics demonstrated not to worsen PD. Olanzepine, risperidone, ziprasidone, and aripiprazole all may worsen parkinsonism.

Usually the patient is amnestic for most of the delirious period and only remembers bits and pieces, as with a bad dream.

While hospitalized, the patient should be mobilized as much as possible. Physical therapy should be ordered as soon as possible to prevent decompensation, which may be permanent in a frail, elderly person. Once acute hospital care is no longer required, some patients should be considered for inpatient rehabilitation at a rehabilitation center.

Since PD patients are subject to pneumonia, particular attention should be paid to the lungs, especially if the patient is deemed

"at risk" for pneumonia by virtue of poor swallowing, weak cough-
ing, immobility, and so on. In these situations it is often wise to order
a respiratory therapy consultation for "chest PT" before a problem
develops. These therapists will clap on the chest for several minutes
each day to help mobilize the sputum and make it easier to cough up.
This opens the airways, making breathing easier and infection less
likely to develop.

Certain medications should be avoided by PD patients.
Metoclopramide (Reglan) which is used for reduced gut motility problems, and prochlorperazine (Compazine), which is used for
nausea, should be used as little as possible, if at all. Prochlorperazine
can be replaced by ondansetron (Zofran). Zofran is quite expensive,
but should only be required for a short period of time. For patients
taking seligiline (Eldepryl), it is recommended that the narcotic pain
medication meperidine (Demerol) not be used because of a possible
interaction.

ADVANCE DIRECTIVES

Durable power of attorney for health care and living wills: It is
important to decide in advance of a life-threatening emergency what
to do about it. This may avoid severe family problems later on. Many
patients have strong feelings about being put on mechanical breathing devices or having a variety of invasive procedures performed.
This issue should be discussed before the emergency and the staff
should be properly directed on the level of intervention the patient
and family want.

Glossary

· ·

Acute: Sudden onset.

AD: See Alzheimer's disease

Affect: Mood as conveyed by face, voice, "body language," appearance, and so on. PD patients are often thought to be depressed because their affect is one of depression. They have a depressed facial expression, soft voice, and flexed body position. They also move slowly.

Akathisia: The syndrome of restlessness, relieved to some degree by standing and moving about. Unlike restless legs syndrome, this is present all day, not just at night.

Akinesia: Absence or reduction of movement. PD patients tend to not blink, swallow, or move as much as normal people. This leads to the "staring" due to reduced blinking, the drooling, due to reduced swallowing, and the general "statuesque" quality of PD patients. They tend to sit or stand in one posture and not move.

Akinetic: Having akinesia.

Alzheimer's disease (AD): A progressive disease that destroys memory and other important mental functions. It's the most common cause of dementia.

Amnesia: Impaired memory.

Amnestic: Having amnesia.

Anhedonia: Inability to enjoy or have pleasure.

Anterograde amnesia: Amnesia from a certain time forward.

Anticholinergic: A term for a family of medications that block the action of acetylcholine, an important chemical naturally found in the brain. These medications include benztropine (Cogentin), trihexiphenidyl (Artane), procyclidine (Kemadrin), and biperiden (Akineton).

Antipsychotic: A drug that treats psychotic symptoms. These drugs are most commonly used to treat schizophrenia but may also be helpful in treating hallucinations and delusions caused in PD patients by their PD medications.

Anxiety: Nervousness.

Anxiety disorders: A collection of several different syndromes, each of which includes increased nervousness.

Anxiolytic: A drug that treats anxiety ("lytic" means "breaks").

Apathy: Not caring, having reduced emotions, and lessened interest.

Aphasia: From "a" meaning without and "phasia" meaning language; a language disorder out of proportion to other impairments of thinking and memory.

Apnea: Not breathing.

Apraxia: Inability to perform a motor act despite having normal strength and coordination; for example, a patient tries to touch his finger to his nose but makes a fist instead. The "motor programs" for the two acts have gotten confused in the brain. Even though the patient is physically able to move the hand to the nose, he cannot actually will the act to occur.

Aspiration: Something swallowed that ends up "going the wrong way" into the lungs. This may cause pneumonia.

Baseline: The condition the patient is usually in, which forms the basis for comparing any change. A patient may improve from his baseline, as with starting a new medication for the PD, or he may worsen, as when having a side effect.

Bonnet's syndrome: A term used to describe elderly people who develop visual hallucinations as a result of increasingly impaired vision. These patients are otherwise normal, without memory, thinking, or behavior problems. This is not at all related to PD, but may explain an occasional PD patient who develops visual hallucinations, particularly if the person is not taking any PD medications.

Bradykinesia: Slowness of movement. Bradykinesia is often the most disabling of the various problems that PD patients have. The loss of dexterity in buttoning, using a zipper, cutting food, all are part-and-parcel of the slowness. The fact that it takes so much longer to dress, bathe, write, balance the checkbook, and so on, reduces the amount of work a PD patient can accomplish.

Bradyphrenia: Slowness of thinking. Some PD patients take longer to respond to questions or to solve problems. In some cases this may be due to slowness in speech, but it may also be due to a problem with actually solving the problem or responding to the request. Patients will be able to state whether the slowness is a speech or response problem or whether it is a thinking problem. Bradyphrenia has no known treatment.

Capgras syndrome: This is also called the syndrome of reduplication. People believe that objects and even people have been replaced by exact copies. The wedding ring with an engraved message, the prescription eyeglasses, the handwritten notes, even one's spouse, have all been replaced by exact copies.

Central sleep apnea: This is a very uncommon syndrome in which the brain tells the body not to breathe.

Cholinesterase inhibitors: These medications increase the amount of acetylcholine in the brain. They work by blocking the system that breaks down the acetylcholine. This is the opposite of the anticholinergic drugs. These medications are used primarily in Alzheimer's disease, but are also used in other dementing illnesses, including PD. These medications may help with memory, concentration and mood. These drugs are donepezil (Aricept), galantamine (Reminyl), and rivastigmine (Exelon).

Cognition: The ability to understand and solve problems; this is a general term meaning "thinking," which is separate from memory.

Compulsion: An urge to do something over and over, such as cleaning one's hands repetitively or checking that the door is locked several times.

Confabulate: Make up. Confabulations, unlike lies, are created to fill a memory void rather than to fool another person. The patient believes the statements are true. Confabulations can be bizarre, but usually are ordinary, everyday sorts of experiences. "What did you do yesterday?" "I went to the ballgame," even though the patient is bedbound in the nursing home.

Confusion: A general term meaning disoriented with impaired memory and impaired thinking skills. This may refer to a long-standing chronic condition, a progressive problem, or an acute change. Acute confusional states are the same as a delirium.

Control population: A group of people who are used for comparison purposes.

Cortex: The outer mantle of the brain. A major location for language and emotions.

Cortical: Referring to the cortex.

Cortical dementia: In understanding dementia, the term "cortical" refers to brain functions that are thought to be centered in the brain's cortex or outer mantle. The primary functions considered "cortical" are language and praxis, the ability to perform an action that the brain "knows" how to perform.

DLB: See Dementia with Lewy bodies

DDS (dopamine dysregulation syndrome): A condition in which patients behave as if addicted to L-Dopa, craving the drug even when it causes side effects.

Delirious: A mental state in which the patient has diminished attention and is easily distracted. The patient is usually disoriented, not knowing perhaps where he is, what time of day it is, what month or year it is, who is in the nearby environment, and what is going on around him. The patient frequently misunderstands explanations for things, has peculiar interpretations for events, and is irrational or irritable in a manner that is atypical for the patient when he is "normal."

Delusion: A false or irrational belief. While delusions can be "benign," or not bothersome, they usually are very bothersome. Believing that the grandchildren visited in the morning, although they live 3,000 miles away and are known to be at their own home, is a benign delusion. Thinking that the spouse is having an affair, or that the neighbors are poisoning the water supply, are harmful and paranoid delusions.

Dementia: A decline in intellectual function leading to some degree of social impairment as the result of reduced memory or problem-solving abilities.

Dementia with Lewy bodies (DLB): The second most common type of progressive dementia after Alzheimer's disease, causes a progressive decline in mental abilities. An indicator of Lewy body dementia may be significant fluctuations in alertness and attention, which may include daytime drowsiness or periods of staring into space. And, like PD, DLB can result in rigid muscles, slowed movement and tremors. In DLB, abnormal round structures, called Lewy bodies, develop in regions of the brain involved in thinking and movement.

Depression: A collection of several symptoms, with either sadness or an inability to feel pleasure being a central feature. Depression also may include fatigue, poor sleeping, weight loss or weight gain, soft voice, and irritability.

Disinhibited: Loss of inhibition, becoming unconstrained by usual social norms and therefore doing things that would be considered embarrassing by others.

Dopamine: Shorthand for di-ortho-phenylalanine, the chemical that is reduced in PD.

Dopamine agonist: A drug that has chemical properties similar to dopamine.

Dopamine antagonist: A drug that blocks the effect of dopamine. These drugs make motor function worse in people with PD.

Dopamine dysregulation syndrome: See DDS.

Dyskinesia: An abnormal movement, usually caused by L-Dopa or dopamine agonists, which is usually jerky or writhing. It is different from a tremor, which is a very regular, unchanging, back-and-forth type of movement.

Encephalopathy: A condition of decreased or altered level of alertness, usually associated with a degree of confusion. This term can be used to mean delirium, if there is a recent change in behavior, but also can refer to someone who has old brain changes that haven't changed, as in an adult who was born with cerebral palsy.

Etiology: Cause, as in, the etiology of his coma was a brain tumor.

Fatigue: A sense of lack of energy, which is different from feeling sleepy. This is a common problem in PD.

Hallucination: A sensation that is not based on any stimulus. Hallucinations need to be distinguished from illusions and dreams. Hallucinations may occur in each of the special senses: vision, hearing, taste, smell, and touch. If a person sees something that is fairly clear but disappears when approached, it is a hallucination. This is different from seeing a form in a shadow, or seeing something that is unclear that is first thought to be one thing then is more clearly seen for what it actually is. One can taste food, or smell an odor that is not present, or even feel things moving on the skin although nothing can be seen.

Hypertension: High blood pressure.

Hypnotic: A drug to help a patient fall asleep.

Hypotension: Low blood pressure. This is what causes fainting.

ICD (impulse control disorder): A condition, most often caused by dopamine agonists (pramipexole, ropinerole, bromocriptine, rotigotine, and lisuride) in which people develop uncontrolled urges to perform some activity on a compulsive basis. The most common of such behaviors are gambling, hypersexuality, spending excessive amounts of money, surfing the Internet, and so on.

Ictal: Sudden onset of a neurological problem.

Illusion: A distorted perception. Unlike a hallucination, an illusion is based on something that is really present, but is misinterpreted. A shadow is mistaken for a dog. A fire hydrant seen at a far distance is thought to be a child on a bicycle. A passing truck is heard as a shouting parade. Illusions are very common, particularly visual illusions. These are "abnormal" only when they become excessively common and interfere with normal function.

Impulse control disorder: See ICD.

Inner tremor: The sensation of a part of the body having a tremor when it is not actually moving. This frequently affects parts of the body that do not develop tremors, such as the chest or neck.

Leukoaraiosis: A term used in CT scans to describe changes in the white matter of the brain that are the same as small vessel ischemic disease (SVID) (see entry). The white matter, which is made up of fibers connecting one part of the brain to another begin to deteriorate.

Lewy body: An abnormal ball of proteins that is found in certain areas of the brain in people with PD. These are contained within the brain cells and can only be seen under a microscope. Their presence is usually a sign of PD.

Motor: Having to do with movement or muscles. Motor dysfunction refers to the slowness, stiffness, and other problems PD patients have with their mobility. This may include speech problems, which are due to poor coordination of the muscles involved in speaking, drooling, which is due to reduced swallowing, eye tearing, due to reduced blinking and therefore drying of the eyes and then a tearing response, and so on.

MRI (magnetic resonance imaging): A technique for producing an extremely detailed picture of the brain, better than a CT scan, and without any radiation. It is not very useful in PD because the abnormalities of PD cannot be seen on an MRI.

Narcolepsy: A neurological condition that appears in younger people, not related to PD, in which the patient requires large amounts of sleep and is usually sleepy all the time.

Neurodegenerative: A "neurodegenerative" disorder is a nervous system disorder that worsens, or degenerates, over time. We frequently talk of "disease progression," which also means disease worsening, also known as "advancing" disease. We thus use words that mean the opposite, "advance" and "decline," "progress" and "degenerate" interchangeably. PD always worsens with time.

Neuron: A nervous system cell that is involved in carrying information.

Neurotransmitter: A chemical that a brain neuron secretes to communicate with the next brain cell. Each cell produces primarily one neurotransmitter, but there are many different ones in the normal brain.

Nocebo: An inert substance that causes negative effects. A "sugar pill" which might make someone feel better (placebo) might also cause side effects and thus be a "negative" placebo.

Obstructive sleep apnea: This is very common. The muscles in the throat relax too much so that the windpipe collapses and blocks the flow of air into the lungs. As a result the patient can't breathe. As the body's carbon dioxide rises, the drive to breathe becomes strong enough to overcome the collapsed airway, which produces a snoring sound. Obstructive sleep apnea is common in PD, but is also common in the general population, especially among obese smokers.

Orientation: The ability of the patient to know where she is, what the date and time are, what she is doing, and what the people around her are doing.

Orthostatic hypotension: Low blood pressure that develops on standing up. This is quite common in PD and leads to many falls.

Pallidotomy: Making a small hole ("-otomy") in a small structure, deep in the brain, which is called the "globus pallidum."

Paranoia: A belief that others are trying to harm someone close to the patient, or the patient herself.

Pathological gambling: Gambling to the point of potential financial or social harm.

Phobia: Irrational fear.

Placebo: A "dummy" medicine; an inert substance put into a pill so that doctors and patients can't tell if they are receiving the active study drug or not.

Postictal state: The condition that exists after the acute problem.

Premorbid: Before the illness.

Pseudo-dementia: Having memory or thinking impairment due to depression, anxiety, pain, or medication effects.

Pseudo-depression: Looking depressed but not actually being depressed, a "false" depression. Many PD patients are thought to be depressed because of their appearance, but they are not really depressed.

Psychomotor retardation: Slowing of movement and thought, a very common problem seen both in nondepressed PD patients as well as in people with depression who do not have PD.

Punding: Senseless repetitive activities, usually taking objects apart and putting them back together, but also includes endless recataloging of collections, repetitive checking of sums, needless reordering of files, and so on.

REM: Rapid eye movement.

REM sleep: The dream portion of sleep, during which normal people are paralyzed except for their breathing and their eye movements. The eyes move, as if following the action in the dream.

REM sleep behavior disorder (RBD): A syndrome in which people are occasionally not paralyzed during dream (REM) sleep, so that they act out their dreams, even though they are asleep. This affects men five times more commonly than women. It affects about 30% of men with PD.

Restless legs syndrome: A common condition in which people feel uncomfortable sensations in their legs, particularly at night when they lay down to go to sleep. They get relief by moving.

Retrograde memory loss: Loss of memory affecting the most recent memories the greatest and the most distant memories the least.

Rigidity: Stiffness. In PD the joints, even when relaxed, resist movement. Patients sometimes feel stiff, but not always. If you move the wrist, elbow, or head of a normal person who is relaxed, the limb moves as if it is on a well-oiled joint. In PD the movement encounters resistance, as if the patient is tensing the muscles on purpose to prevent the movement or slow it down. This resistance is part of the disease and may contribute to the stooped posture and other changes in appearance that occur in PD sedation sleepiness.

Sedative: A drug to help a patient calm down or sleep.

Sleep apnea: Not breathing during sleep. Actually the patient only stops breathing for a period of time or else he would die. The long breath-holding interferes with sleep quality and makes the patient very sleepy during the day. There are two forms of sleep apnea, obstructive and central (see definitions).

Sleep architecture: There are several stages of sleep, and normal people have a relatively similar profile for when they enter each stage and how long they remain in each stage. There are many ways to disturb the "normal" sleep cycle, including altered sleep habits, alcohol and other medications, and a variety of neurologic disorders, including PD.

Small vessel ischemic disease (SVID): A term used in describing changes in the white matter of the brain seen on brain MRI. These changes look like white patches and may be difficult to distinguish from small strokes. They are caused by slowly developing changes in the brain's blood vessels during which the small arteries become narrowed and stiff. As a result of the blood vessel changes, deterioration of the surrounding brain cells occurs, with impairment of the nerve cells' ability to reliably conduct impulses from one part of the brain to another.

Somnolence: Sleepiness.

SSRI (selective serotonin reuptake inhibitor): A class of antidepressant drugs including fluoxetine (Prozac), sertraline (Zoloft), paroxetine (Paxil), and others.

Stroke: Also known as a cerebrovascular accident, a stroke is the loss of brain tissue due to either a blockage of blood flow to a region of the brain or the rupture of a blood vessel in the brain causing a blood clot to form.

Substantia nigra: The part of the brain that is most affected in PD. The term means "black body" because this region of the brain is pigmented so that it looks black to the naked eye.

SVID: See small vessel ischemic disease.

Syndrome: A collection of symptoms that often occur together.

Thalamotomy: Making a small hole ("-otomy") in a region in the middle of the brain called the "thalamus."

Vivid dream: A very realistic dream.

Index

@ indicates a table